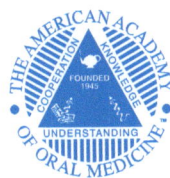

CLINICIAN'S GUIDE

Treatment of Medically Complex Dental Patients

FIFTH EDITION

EDITOR

Thamer M. Musbah, BDS
Assistant professor of Oral Medicine
Department of Oral Health Practice
University of Kentucky College of Dentistry, KY

ASSOCIATE EDITOR

Craig S. Miller, DMD, MS
Professor of Oral Medicine
Department of Oral Health Practice
University of Kentucky College of Dentistry, KY

CONTRIBUTING AUTHORS IN CURRENT EDITON (5TH)

Chizobam Idahosa, DDS
Ying Wai Sia, DDS
Thamer M Musba, BDS

CONTRIBUTING AUTHORS IN CURRENT EDITON (4TH)

Ramesh Balasubramaniam, BDS
Michael Brennan, DDS, MS
Ronald S. Brown, DDS, MS
Richard P. Cohan, AB, DDS, MS, MA, MBA, FAGD
Craig Hatch, DDS, MS
Michaell Huber, DDS
Joseph L Konzelman, DDS
Janet E. Leigh, BDS, DMD
Peter Lockhart, DMD, MS
Andres Pinto, DMD, MPH
John Robinson, DDS
Thomas P. Sollecito, DMD
Eric T. Stoopler, DMD
Martin T. Tyler, BS, DDS, MEd

CONTENTS

American Academy of Oral Medicine
2150 N. 107th St., Suite 205
Seattle, Washington 98133
TEL: (206) 209-5279
EMAIL: info@aaom.com   WEBSITE: www.aaom.com
©2018 American Academy of Oral Medicine

ISBN
print: 978-1-936176-55-7
PDF: 978-1-936176-56-4

Printed in the United States

Notice: The authors and publisher have made every effort to ensure that the patient care recommended herein, including choice of drugs and drug dosages, is in accord with the accepted standard and practice at the time of publication. However, since research and regulation constantly change clinical standards, the reader is urged to check the product information sheet included in the package of each drug, which includes recommended doses, warnings, and contraindications. This is particularly important with new or infrequently used drugs. Any treatment regimen, particularly one involving medication, involves inherent risk that must be weighed on a case-by-case basis against the benefits anticipated. The reader is cautioned that the purpose of this book is to inform and enlighten; the information contained herein is not intended as, and should not be employed as, a substitute for individual diagnosis and treatment.

The fifth edition of this Guide is dedicated to the memory of Jonathan A. Ship, DMD. Dr. Ship was an inspiration to a generation of students, oral medicine residents and colleagues and a revered member of the American Academy of Oral Medicine. His research contributions in geriatric dentistry, xerostomia, Sjögren's syndrome and oral, head and neck cancer will serve the professional community and society for generations. His friendship, guidance, professionalism and laughter are sorely missed by everyone who knew and loved him. Dr. Ship has contributed extensively to earlier versions of this Guide.

ABOUT THE AMERICAN ACADEMY OF ORAL MEDICINE (AAOM): The AAOM is a 501c6; nonprofit organization founded in 1945 as the American Academy of Dental Medicine and took its current name in 1966. The members of the American Academy of Oral Medicine include an internationally recognized group of health care professionals and experts concerned with the oral health care of patients who have complex medical conditions, oral mucosal disorders, and / or chronic orofacial pain. Oral Medicine is the field of dentistry concerned with the oral health care of medically complex patients and with the diagnosis and non-surgical management of medically-related disorders or conditions affecting the oral and maxillofacial region.

AMERICAN ACADEMY OF ORAL MEDICINE

MISSION:

1. To promote the study and dissemination of knowledge of the medical aspects of dentistry while serving the best interests of the public.

2. To promote the highest standards of care in the diagnosis and treatment of oral conditions that are not responsive to conventional dental or oral maxillofacial surgical procedures.

3. To provide an avenue of referral for dental practitioners who have patients with severe, life- threatening medical disorders or complex diagnostic problems involving the oral and maxillofacial region that require ongoing nonsurgical management.

4. To improve the quality of life of patients with medically related oral disease.

5. To foster increased understanding and cooperation between medical and dental professions.

6. To obtain American Dental Association recognition of oral medicine as a specialty.

The Academy achieves these goals by holding national meetings annually; by presenting lectures, workshops, and seminars; by sponsorship of the American Board of Oral Medicine; by the editorship of the Oral Medicine Section of *Oral Surgery, Oral Medicine, Oral Pathology, Oral Radiology*, and *Endodontics*; and by publishing monographs and position papers on timely subjects relating to oral medicine.

The presented information is based on current knowledge and accepted standards of practice. Following the guidelines set forth in this monograph may not ensure successful management of every patient. This monograph represents a consensus of the editors and authors and not necessarily the private views of any individual.

All brand name medications may have patents, service marks, trademarks, or registered trademarks and are the property of their respective companies.

This Clinician's Guide is another AAOM educational service.
Other Clinician's Guides available from the Academy include:

Tobacco Cessation
Oral Health in Geriatric Patients
Pharmacology in Dental Medicine
Chronic Orofacial Pain
Treatment of Common Oral Conditions
Salivary Gland & Chemosensory Disorders 1/e

Introduction

Systemic health is often related to oral health. Many systemic diseases (i.e., cancer, hypertension, cardio-vascular disease, diabetes, leukemia, gastrointestinal disorders, osteoporosis, autoimmune diseases, human immunodeficiency virus [HIV], and other infectious diseases) are often manifested in the oral cavity. In addition, some of these conditions and the therapies used to treat them have effects on the teeth and mouth. For those reasons, it is important for dentists to know about their patients' medical conditions before treating them and to understand which diseases manifest themselves in the oral cavity. It is equally important for physicians to understand what their patients' oral health can reveal about their overall health and potential for disease. This guide-book outlines what dental practitioners should know when managing patients with certain conditions, such as cardiovascular disease and arthritis, and/or who are being treated with certain medications, such as chemotherapy agents, as well as how dentists can help detect underlying undiagnosed or poorly controlled medical conditions to better serve patients. Today, considerable attention and research are focused on the association between oral infection and systemic disease, how dental treatment can affect systemic conditions, and, conversely, how systemic diseases and their treatments can affect the oral cavity.

Additionally, new diagnostic methods are emerging that use oral tissues or fluids for the diagnosis of systemic conditions. Dentists play a key role in screening for undiagnosed conditions, such as cancer, hypertension, diabetes, leukemia, gastrointestinal disorders, osteoporosis, autoimmune diseases, HIV, and other infectious diseases.

Virtually any medical condition may affect dental treatment and vice versa. Dentists should establish the nature and physical status of these conditions in their patients and approach the comprehensive care of patients in a manner to ensure their overall welfare. Outlined here are some of the more common medical conditions, how to recognize and assess them, and proper dental management.

For the Editors
Thamer M. Musbah, BDS
Craig S. Miller, DMD, MS

Standard Abbreviations

I	One	Prn	as needed (pro re nata)
ii	Two	Q	Every
iii	Three	q2h	every 2 hours
a	Before	q4h	every 4 hours
ac	before meals (ante cibum)	q6h	every 6 hours
ad lib	as desired (ad libitum)	q8h	every 8 hours
asap	as soon as possible	q12h	every 12 hours
AAOM	American Academy of Oral Medicine	Qam	every morning
bid	twice a day (bis in die)	Qd	every day (quaque die)
btl	Bottle	Qhs	every bedtime
c	With	Qid	four times a day (quarter in die)
cap	Capsule	Qod	every other day
CBC	complete blood count	Qpm	every evening
CDC	U. S. Center for Disease Control and Prevention	qsad	add a sufficient quantity to equal
crm	Cream	qwk	every week
disp	dispense on a prescription label	RAS	recurrent aphthous stomatitis
elix	Elixir	RAU	recurrent aphthous ulcer
FDA	U.S. Food and Drug Administration	RBC	red blood cell count
g	Gram	RHL	recurrent herpes labialis
gtt	Drop	RIH	recurrent intraoral herpes
h	Hour	Rx	Prescription
hs	at bedtime	s	Without
HSV	herpes simplex virus	Sig	patient dosing instructions on prescription label
IU	international units	Sol	Solution
IV	Intravenous	SPF	sun protection factor
L	Liter	stat	Immediately
liq	Liquid	Syr	Syrup
loz	Lozenge	Tab	Tablet
mg	Milligram	tbsp	Tablespoon
min	Minute	Tid	three times a day (ter in die)
mL	Milliliter	Top	Topical
NaF	sodium fluoride	Tsp	Teaspoon

Standard Abbreviations (continued)

Oint	Ointment	U	Unit
OTC	over-the-counter	ut dict	as directed (ut dictum)
Oz	Ounce	UV	Ultraviolet
P	After	Visc	Viscous
Pc	after meals	VZV	varicella-zoster virus
PABA	para-aminobenzoic acid	WBC	white blood cell count
PHN	postherpetic neuralgia	Wk	Week
PLT	platelet count	Yr	Year
Po	by mouth (per os)	Zn	Zinc

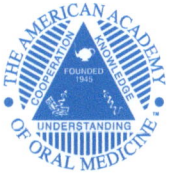

1 Cardiovascular Disease

CARDIOVASCULAR DISEASE: GENERAL RISK ASSESSMENT

Many dental patients report a history of cardiovascular disease(s). Other patients may present with signs and/or symptoms that are highly suggestive of cardiovascular disease(s). Also, a cardiac emergency can occur in the dental office. The victim of the cardiac emergency may or may not have identified cardiovascular disease. Therefore, the dentist must be prepared to manage the oral health care needs of patients with cardiovascular disease(s). Patient management may include a consultation with the physician to determine the patient's cardiac status prior to initiating any definitive dental treatment. See Table 1-1 for risk predictors for cardiovascular disease. See Table 1-2 for general critical management guidelines. See Table 1-3 for general considerations.

THE KNOWN CARDIAC PATIENT

Hypertension
- Abnormal elevation of the arterial blood pressure
- Increasing prevalence owing to the increase in the older population
- Hypertension (HTN) usually has no symptoms
- HTN is a major risk factor for end-organ damage: heart, kidney, brain, eyes
- HTN, if untreated, shortens life by 10 to 20 years
- Based on JNC 8 2014 Guidlines
  - 30% of individuals with HTN are unaware they have the condition
  - 59% of individuals with HTN are being treated for the condition
  - Only 34% of individuals with HTN have their blood pressure controlled to current goals.
- Based on the 2017 Guidelines the prevalence of hypertension is expected to increase substantially

See section on hypertension.

PROSTHETIC HEART VALVES
Patients pending surgery to replace a cardiac valve(s):

- Comprehensive dental evaluation
- Remove all sources of active dental disease: caries, periodontal/pulpal pathology, non-restorable teeth

Patients with prosthetic heart valves:

- Higher risk for developing infective endocarditis (IE); accordingly follow American Heart Association (AHA) guidelines for antimicrobial prophylaxis
- Anticoagulant therapy: Vitamin K anticoagulant, International Normalized Ratio (INR) should be 2.0 to 3.5. Ensure that the INR is in the therapeutic range before performing procedures that result in oral bleeding. Non-vitamin K anticoagulants (Direct Oral Anticoagulant-DOAC) generally do not need to be temporarily interrupted for most invasive oral procedures, however adjunctive local hemostatic measures should be used in these circumstances, when needed.

Prior History of IE
Higher incidence of recurrent endocarditis
- AHA guidelines for antimicrobial prophylaxis
- Multiple episodes of IE increase likelihood of morbidity and mortality.

ORAL HEALTH CONSIDERATIONS
- It is important that this individual have optimal oral health to decrease bacteremia from daily activities such as chewing, tooth brushing, and flossing.

See section on IE.

Table 1–1: Risk Predictors*

Major Risk Predictors

1. Unstable coronary syndrome
   - Myocardial infarction (MI) within 1 month
   - Unstable angina pectoris
2. Decompensated heart failure
   - Congestive heart failure resulting in limited normal daily activities
3. Severe valvular disease
4. Significant arrhythmias

Intermediate Risk Predictors

1. Stable angina pectoris
2. Previous MI 1 month or longer
3. Compensated heart failure
4. Diabetes mellitus (particularly type 1)
5. Renal insufficiency

Minor Risk Predictors

1. Advanced age
2. Atrial fibrillation
3. Low (poor) functional capacity (see MET note below)
4. History of stroke
5. Uncontrolled systemic hypertension (>180/110 mm Hg)

Patient: Functional Capacity

1 MET: dress; eat; use toilet; walk indoors around the house; perform light housework such as dusting or washing dishes; walk a block on level ground at 2–3 mph

4 METs: climb a flight of stairs or walk up a hill; walk on level ground at 4 mph; run a short distance; perform heavy work such as moving or lifting heavy furniture, scrubbing floors; participate in moderate activities such as golfing, dancing, throwing a ball

10 METs: participate in strenuous sports such as swimming, singles tennis, football, and basketball

The functional capacity of the patient correlates well with the patient's ability to undergo the stresses associated with comprehensive dental care and is expressed in terms of metabolic equivalents (METs):

Poor < 4 METs

Moderate 4–7 METs

Good 7–10 METs

Excellent > 10 METs

Increased cardiovascular risk associated with noncardiac procedures to include dental procedures

Table 1–2: General Critical Management Guidelines

1. Be aware of the increased risk of morbidity and mortality inherent in cardiovascular disease.

2. Update the medical history at each appointment, paying particular attention to disease severity, previous cardiac surgery, or any recent changes in signs and symptoms.

   a. Assess for the presence of risk predictors of increased cardiovascular risk associated with noncardiac procedures.

   b. Carefully observe for signs/symptoms indicative of a change in the status of the cardiovascular disease:
   - Pallor, cyanosis, peripheral edema, dyspnea, rales, obesity, tremor, anxiety
   - Elevated blood pressure
   - Rapid or abnormal pulse

3. The patient's medications will provide clues to the severity of the disease and help identify those at risk for side effects and possible drug interactions when prescribing medication(s).

4. Carefully observe for signs/symptoms of undiagnosed cardiovascular disease.

5. Prevention and control of oral infections are particularly important in this patient population.

6. The control of stress and prevention of pain are important to minimize endogenous release of catecholamines.

   a. Early afternoon dental appointments are preferable.

   b. Stress reduction protocols as warranted.

7. Consultation with the patient's physician may be indicated to determine the presence of cardiac abnormalities or conditions that require special management recommendations.

Table 1–3: General Considerations

1. Limited dental care:
  • Dental prophylaxis
  • Simple restorative
  • Periodontal
  • Endodontic procedures
  • Routine simple extraction
 	
2. Emergency dental care: the benefit received by intervention outweighs the risk of complications associated with the patient's cardiovascular status. The dental procedures may include pain relief, treatment of infection, and hemostasis:
  • Simple I&D
  • Induction of hemostasis
  • The use of a vasoconstrictor in local anesthesia is advisable to improve the profundity and duration of the anesthesia.
Exceptions are noted in the specific protocols below.
 	
3. Patient on coumarin anticoagulant therapy: monitor with INR. Therapeutic goals for INR vary according to condition (range = 2 to 3.5).
  a. Verify INR on day of treatment
    • Oral surgical procedures generally tolerable if INR is < 3.5
    • Minimize trauma
    • Application of local hemostatic agents
    • Placement of sutures, if applicable
  b. For more extensive surgical procedures or for conditions in which the therapeutic INR target is >3.5:
    • Coordinate with physician to lower INR <3.5
Only the physician should adjust the anticoagulant dose.
 	
4. Implanted pacemakers or implanted cardioconverter devices (ICDs)
  • Electrical medical/dental devices may interfere with function of pacemaker or ICD.
  • Potential risk with electrosurgery unit; ***avoid use***
  • No risk noted with amalgamator, electric pulp tester, curing lights, electric toothbrush, dental unit/light, sonic scaler, endodontic ultrasonic instrument, or radiographic unit
 	
I & D = Incision & Drainage; INR = international normalized ratio; MET = metabolic equivalent.

Congenital Heart Disease
- Atrial septal defect
- Ventricular septal defect
- Complete atrioventricular canal
- Aortic stenosis/insufficiency
- Coarctation of the aorta
- Pulmonary valve stenosis
- Tetralogy of Fallot
- Truncus arteriosus
- Transposition of the great arteries
- Higher risk for IE
- AHA guidelines for antimicrobial prophylaxis

ISCHEMIC HEART DISEASE/ANGINA PECTORIS

Ischemic heart disease (IHD) is indicative of cardiac diseases that result in an imbalance of the limited myocardial oxygen supply and the excessive myocardial oxygen demand.

- Symptomatic IHD is angina pectoris: increased risk for developing acute myocardial infarction. This is a major risk predictor for a cardiovascular event while performing noncardiovascular procedures.
- Stable IHD/angina pectoris is an intermediate risk predictor.
  - Stable angina = chest pain that does not vary by frequency, onset or variability.
- Determine the patient's functional capacity and vital signs.

ANGINA PECTORIS

Definition

Angina pectoris is a clinical term that refers to a transient chest pain/discomfort of moderate intensity that results from myocardial ischemia.

Etiology

Coronary artery arteriosclerosis or atherosclerotic obstruction of one or more of the coronary arteries results in a transient myocardial demand in excess of the available oxygen supply from the coronary vessels.

- Exercise, stress, or exertion may produce this increase in oxygen demand.
- The end result is pain.

Clinical Presentation

Exertional or stress-related substernal pressure, tightness, or moderate discomfort that is relieved by rest.

- The sensation of numbness or tingling may radiate to the shoulders, arms, jaws, and/or throat.

Table 1–4: Specific Management Protocols: Considerations*

1. Patient with minor or intermediate risk predictor(s) for cardiovascular risk: BP < 180/< 110 mm Hg and normal pulse and > 4 MET functional capacity
   - Comprehensive dental care
   - Routine medical referral as warranted for medical management.

2. Patient with minor or intermediate risk predictor(s) for cardiovascular risk: BP < 180/< 110 mm Hg and normal pulse and < 4 MET functional capacity
   - Necessary limited dental care
   - Do not exceed 0.051 mg of epinephrine (≈3 Carpules)

3. Patient with minor or intermediate risk predictor(s) of cardiovascular risk: BP > 180/> 110 mm Hg and/or abnormal pulse
   - Emergency dental treatment
   - *If patient is symptomatic with cardiovascular signs and symptoms: immediate referral for medical evaluation and treatment*
   - If patient is asymptomatic: routine referral for medical management

4. Patient with major risk predictor(s) of cardiovascular risk and clinical signs and symptoms:
   - Emergency dental care
   - Avoid epinephrine use
   - *Immediate referral for medical evaluation and treatment*

BP = blood pressure; MET = metabolic equivalent.
*Refer to Table 1–1.

- The most common areas of radiating pain are the left shoulder and down the medial surface of the left arm. This presentation is more common in men. Women may have atypical presentation.

Refer to specific management protocols: Table 1-4.

ORAL HEALTH CARE CONSIDERATIONS
- Stable angina: routine dental care: limited to patients with stable angina
- Sedative medication prior to stressful dental procedures if indicated
- Appointments: short afternoon appointments with minimal stress

- Monitor blood pressure and pulse at each appointment
- Acceptable dose levels of local anesthetic/epinephrine
  - Should not exceed 0.051 mg: equivalent to three 1.7 mL carpules of 2% lidocaine with 1:100,000 epinephrine
  - Avoid using retraction cord impregnated with epinephrine

ACUTE MYOCARDIAL INFARCTION
Definition
Irreversible myocardial damage and necrosis resulting from prolonged ischemic injury.

Complications from acute MI:
- Conduction defects/arrhythmias
- Myocardial dysfunction/ heart failure
- Mitral valve regurgitation

Etiology
A pronounced decrease in myocardial perfusion produced by (1) atherosclerosis, (2) vasospasm, or (3) thrombotic occlusion of the coronary arteries will result in myocardial infarction.

Clinical Presentation
Severe, prolonged substernal or chest pain that may be accompanied by *dyspnea*, *nausea*, or *vomiting*.
- The pain may radiate to the shoulders, arms, and/or jaws.
- A common patient reaction is denial of a cardiac arrest.
- The patient insists that the pain is gastric in origin.
- The patient has an overwhelming sense of impending doom.

Post-MI cardiac performance depends on the extent of myocardial muscle survival.

Current medical practices make it possible to quickly assess the patient's physical status after their MI and to determine the patient's ability to undergo dental procedures. However, it is recommended that post-MI patients do not have elective dental procedures for at least 1 month after their attack.

ORAL HEALTH CONSIDERATIONS
Acute MI: 1 month or greater
- Consultation with physician to determine patient's post-MI status
  1. Stable patients: minimal cardiac muscle damage; can perform routine dental treatment

2. Severe cardiac muscle damage:
   - Emergency dental treatment
   - Dental team should be on alert and prepared to react to a cardiac emergency occurring during the dental treatment

See section on the emergency cardiac patient.
- Short, nonstressful afternoon appointments
- Patients may be taking anticoagulant/antiplatelet medications to prevent thromboembolic events
  1. If patient takes coumarin, ensure that the INR is in the therapeutic range, 2.0 to 3.5.
- Monitor blood pressure and pulse before, during, and after dental procedures
- Acceptable dose levels of local anesthetic/epinephrine for the patient with minimal cardiac muscle damage
  - Should not exceed 0.051 mg — equivalent to three 1.7 mL Carpules of 2% lidocaine with 1:100,000 epinephrine
  - Avoid using retraction cord impregnated with epinephrine

Acute MI beyond 1 month
- Consultation with physician to determine patient's post-MI status
- Routine dental treatment can be performed
- Nonstressful afternoon appointments
- Patients may be taking anticoagulant/antiplatelet medications to prevent thromboembolic events
  1. If patient takes coumarin, ensure that the INR is in the therapeutic range, 2.0 to 3.0.
- Acceptable dose levels of local anesthetic/epinephrine
  1. Should not exceed 0.051 mg — equivalent to three 1.7 mL Carpules of 2% lidocaine with 1:100,000 epinephrine
  2. Avoid using retraction cord impregnated with epinephrine

ARRHYTHMIAS
Electrocardiographic evidence of abnormal atrial or ventricular electrical activity may produce symptoms and cardiovascular compromise

ORAL HEALTH CONSIDERATIONS
- The type and severity of the arrhythmia will determine your management.
  1. Patients with uncontrolled atrial fibrillation are at increased risk for stroke.
  2. Concomitant coronary artery disease and congestive heart failure place the patient at increased risk.
  3. These are major risk predictors; refer to Table 1-1.

Patients may have a pacemaker or automated implantable cardioconverter defibrillator.
1. Avoid external electromagnetic devices.
   Refer to General Considerations: Table 1-4.

2. AHA does not recommend antimicrobial prophylaxis.

Arrhythmias without significant cardiac disease must be managed with effective anxiety control.
1. Preoperative use of anxiolytics
2. Short appointments

Monitor blood pressure and pulse at each appointment; give special attention to the pulse rate and rhythm.

Patients may be taking a cardiac glycoside (digoxin/digitoxin) and an anticoagulant.

1. Be aware of cardiac glycoside toxicity: anorexia, nausea, vomiting, and visual disturbances (yellow-green)
2. Evaluate coagulation status; INR is within therapeutic range, 2.0 to 3.5
3. Oral adverse side effects: oral ulcerations and xerostomia

CONGESTIVE HEART DISEASE
Congestive heart disease is an advanced stage of impaired heart function with edema and congestion of pulmonary and systemic venous circulation.

ORAL HEALTH CONSIDERATIONS
- Metabolic demand, morbidity, and mortality increase with severity of the disease.
  - Minimize patient stress to decrease cardiac workload.
  - Compensated heart failure (intermediate risk predictor)
    - Routine dental treatment can be performed.
  - Decompensated heart failure (major risk predictor)
    - Emergency dental treatment
- Pulmonary congestion with respiratory distress may develop with patients who are placed in a supine position for extended periods of time.
- Oral side effects of congestive heart failure medications:
  1. Digoxin/digitalis: nausea, vomiting, exaggerated gag reflex
  2. Diuretics: xerostomia, lichenoid drug reaction
  3. Angiotensin-converting enzyme inhibitors: oral ulcerations, altered taste, angioedema

CORONARY ARTERY BYPASS GRAFT/CORONARY ARTERY STENTS

A history of coronary artery bypass graft (CABG) or placement of stents is associated with marked accumulation of atherosclerotic plaques on the walls of the coronary arteries that compromised the delivery of oxygen to support myocardial activity. These intervention procedures have reduced the incidence of angina and improved the patient's prognosis; however, without lifestyle changes (diet, tobacco use, sedentary lifestyle), restenosis is a potential problem.

ORAL HEALTH CONSIDERATIONS
- If patient presents for dental visit prior to the CABG surgery:
  1. Comprehensive dental evaluation
  2. Remove all sources of active dental disease: caries, periodontal/pulpal pathology, nonrestorable teeth

Elective dental treatment should be deferred postsurgery until the patient is medically stable.

Antimicrobial prophylaxis is not recommended after the period of re-endothelialization of the vessels, usually 2 weeks.

HEART TRANSPLANT RECIPIENT

If time permits prior to the transplant surgery:
- Comprehensive dental evaluation
- Remove all sources of active dental disease: caries, periodontal/pulpal pathology, nonrestorable teeth

After the transplant surgery, consultation with the cardiologist is mandatory.

Increased risk for infection and organ rejection Valve degeneration may occur—increased risk for IE.

ORAL HEALTH CONSIDERATIONS
- Immunosuppressive drugs can have adverse oral effects:
  1. Increased potential for infection
  2. Xerostomia
  3. Candidiasis
  4. Increased risk for activation of the latent herpes virus—intraoral herpetic infection
  5. Cyclosporine – may cause gingival overgrowth

| Table 1–5: Signs and Symptoms of Cardiac Disease ||
Sign/Symptom	Cardiovascular Consideration
Elevated blood pressure	Undiagnosed hypertension
Gross obesity	Risk factor for cardiovascular disease
Tobacco use: smoking	Risk factor for cardiovascular disease
Chest pain/pressure/tightness	Myocardial ischemia Angina pectoris Myocardial infarction
Dyspnea/shortness of breath Orthopnea Paroxysmal nocturnal dyspnea Rales – abnormal respiratory sound	Congestive heart failure – Left-sided heart failure
Distended neck veins Ascites Peripheral edema—swollen ankles	Congestive heart failure – Right-sided heart failure
Clubbed fingernails	Congestive heart failure
Nail bed cyanosis	Congenital heart disease
Xerostomia	Side effects of antihypertensive medications
Orthostatic hypotension/ lightheadedness Headache Depression Visual disturbances Palpitations	
Heart murmur	May indicate valvular disease/Risk for congestive heart failure
Arrhythmias	Underlying atherosclerotic heart disease/Conduction abnormalities

PATIENT WITH SIGNS AND SYMPTOMS OF CARDIAC DISEASE

A dental patient may not identify any cardiovascular disease but can present with signs, symptoms, or risk factors suggestive of cardiac disease that can have important implications in the appropriate dental management for these patients (Table 1-5).

Table 1–6: Emergency Management of Angina & Myocardial Infarction
• Stop all dental treatment.
• Evaluate the patient's status.
• Put the patient in the proper position.   – If conscious, an upright (slightly reclined) position is preferred to facilitate normal patient respiration.
• Activate emergency medical system (EMS); call 911.
• Administer nitroglycerin 0.4 mg sublingually, maximum of three doses at 5-minute intervals.
• Confirm that there is no aspirin allergy.
• Administer aspirin (crushed), 325 mg orally.

• Administer oxygen:
  – 4 L/min flow – nasal cannula
  – 6 L/min flow – face mask

• Record and monitor vital signs until the EMS arrives.
• Be prepared to initiate cardiopulmonary resuscitation.

THE EMERGENCY CARDIAC PATIENT

A sudden onset of symptoms listed above in any patient with or without a prior history of cardiovascular disease can indicate a cardiac emergency. Most of the time, there will be a medical history finding identifying the presence of cardiovascular diseases. Every dentist should be prepared to assess the medical event and to provide appropriate emergency medical treatment when indicated. See Table 1-6. Ischemic heart disease can be divided into two categories, symptomatic (Angina pectoris and myocardial infarction) and asymptomatic (silent myocardial ischemia). Often it is difficult for the clinician to be able to distinguish between these conditions based solely on the presenting acute clinical findings. The clinical presentation of asymptomatic ischemic heart disease includes shortness of breath, nausea, diaphoresis and fatigue.

CARDIAC ARREST

Definition

A sudden cessation of normal cardiac function with a disappearance of arterial blood pressure. This denotes either ventricular fibrillation or tachycardia.

• Absence of responsiveness and pulse

Etiology

Myopathy and coronary artery disease with subsequent pathophysiologic complications that produce myocardial scarring, failure of the myocardium, and heart failure.

Table 1–7: Emergency Management of Cardiac Arrest
• Recognize that the patient has lost consciousness.
• Stop all dental treatment.
• Evaluate the patient's physical status.
• Activate the emergency medical system (EMS); call 911.
• Initiate cardiopulmonary resuscitation.
• Evaluate for defibrillation with an automated external defibrillator.
• Continue lifesaving procedures until EMS arrives and takes over the management of the patient.

Clinical Presentation

Respiratory arrest usually precedes cardiac arrest.

- Cardiac arrest results from cessation of circulation and the absence of detectable blood pressure and pulse.
- Seizure may accompany the cardiac arrest.

Emergency Treatment

Institute basic life support immediately.

- Clinical death can readily follow cardiac arrest but may be reversed if properly managed.

HYPERTENSION

Practicing dentists will encounter many patients with undetected or poorly controlled hypertension requiring medical consultation or intervention. See Table 1–8. Failure to detect severe elevations of blood pressure can potentially result in stroke or myocardial infarction.

Benefits of Lowering Blood Pressure

Effective antihypertensive therapy

- Reduces the incidence of stroke by 35 to 40%
- Reduces myocardial infarction by 20 to 25%
- Reduces heart failure by more than 50%

Dental Monitoring

- The new gudlines urges all health care professionals, including dentists, to become actively involved in the detection and prevention of hypertension.

Table 1– 8: ACC/AHA 2017 Classification of Blood Pressure in Adults		
Blood Pressure Classification	Systolic Blood Pressure* (mm Hg)	Diastolic Blood Pressure* (mm Hg)
Normal	< 120	and < 80
Elevated	120–129	and < 80
Stage 1 hypertension	130–139	or 80–89
Stage 2 hypertension	≥140	or ≥ 90
Hypertension Crisis	>180	>120

ACC = American College of Cardiology   AHA = American College of Cardiology

* Treatment determined by highest blood pressure category.

Little JW, Falace DA, Miller CS, Rhodus NL. Dental management of the medically compromised patient. Mosby Elsevier Publ. Co. St. Louis, MO 2007. p. 37.

- Blood pressure readings should be taken on all new patients and for recall patients at every appointment.
- Individuals who are hypertensive should have blood pressure assessed at each visit in which significant dental procedures are accomplished.
- Dentists should thoroughly review the health history and be familiar with all significant past and current medical problems as well as current medications.

Dental Management of Patients with Hypertension
- Measurement of blood pressure and review of the health status should be routine for all patients but particularly for individuals with known hypertension.
- When elevated blood pressure is detected, or a patient is a known hypertensive and the BP is above goal, the patient should be advised and encouraged to see his or her physician.
- Patients presenting for urgent dental care may have elevations of blood pressure. Causes include (1) undetected hypertension, (2) inadequate treatment, (3) poor patient compliance with physician recommendations, (4) expense of medical care or medications, and (5) avoidance of medication use owing to complications.

Patients with Well-Controlled Hypertension or with Stage 1 Hypertension
- Patients with well-controlled or stage 1 hypertension are good candidates for all dental procedures.
- Moderate hypertension is not an independent risk factor for perioperative cardiovascular complications.
- Risk assessment is essential for all patients, especially those in which complex or surgical procedures are anticipated.

- Sedation with nitrous oxide or an anxiolytic agent is appropriate for anxious individuals.

Use of Vasoconstrictors in Anesthetic Solutions
- Two to three cartridges of lidocaine with 1:100,000 epinephrine (approximately 0.024 to 0.051 mg epinephrine) is considered safe in ambulatory patients with all but the most severe cardiovascular disease.
- Retraction cord containing epinephrine should be avoided.

Patients with Stage 2 Hypertension
- Repeat blood pressure determinations to confirm initial findings and advise the patient to see his or her physician.
- Emergency care may be accomplished as long as SBP is < 180 mm Hg and DBP is < 110 mm Hg.

Patients with SBP > 180 mm Hg and/or DBP > 110 mm Hg
- Elevated blood pressure (SBP 180–209 mm Hg or DBP 110–119 mm Hg) should be referred for immediate medical evaluation.
- Patients with markedly elevated blood pressure and acute target organ damage such as encephalopathy, myocardial infarction, and unstable angina require hospitalization.
- Patients with marked blood pressure elevation without acute target organ damage usually can be managed by immediate combination oral antihypertensive therapy.

Complications of Hypertensive Treatment
Many antihypertensive drugs can cause potential adverse

Table 1–9: Adverse Reactions From Antihypertensive Drugs	
Condition/Finding	**Comment**
Orthostatic hypotension	Particularly older individuals on multiple cardiovascular medications if they attempt to immediately stand upright after being placed in a reclining/supine position for prolonged periods of time
Hypokalemia	Low potassium is a potential side effect of thiazide diuretics and prolonged use of loop diuretics. Hypokalemia can produce ventricular arrhythmias.
Xerostomia	Many medications including central α-agonists and other centrally acting drugs, β-adrenergic blockers, α-adrenergic blocking agents, diuretics, angiotensin converting-enzyme inhibitors, and calcium channel blockers. The likelihood of xerostomia grows as the number of medications with xerostomic potential increases.
Gingival overgrowth	Enlargement of the gingiva is possible with most of the calcium channel blockers, but the majority of cases reported are associated with the use of nifedipine.
Lichenoid reactions	Several cardiovascular medications (thiazides, methyldopa, propranolol, angiotensin-converting enzyme inhibitors, furosemide, spironolactone, and labetalol) have the potential to result in lesions that are indistinguishable from oral lichen planus
Cough/loss of taste	Angiotensin-converting enzyme inhibitors
Scalded lip syndrome	Angiotensin-converting enzyme inhibitors
Angioedema	Angiotensin-converting enzyme inhibitors

reactions that dental clinicians should be aware of and recognize. Table 1–9 is a summary table of the more common of these.

INFECTIVE ENDOCARDITIS:
Definition
Infective endocarditis (IE) is an acute or subacute infection of the valvular or endothelial surfaces of the heart.

Etiology
In the susceptible patient, platelet or fibrin vegetations develop on previously altered cardiac surfaces. Invasive dental procedures can introduce bacteria into the bloodstream, where colonization can occur on the vegetations.

Clinical Presentation
IE may present as an acute, subacute, or chronic disease. Common early symptoms of subacute IE include unexplained low-grade fever, malaise, anemia, weight loss, and joint pains. These symptoms may persist for weeks prior to the diagnosis being made. As IE progresses, dyspnea, orthopnea, a pathologic heart murmur, embolic phenomena, stroke, congestive heart failure, renal failure, meningitis, and multiple manifestations of disseminated immune-mediated vasculitis may be noted.

Diagnosis
The two major criteria for the diagnosis of IE are positive blood cultures for organisms typical of the disease and echocardiographic evidence of cardiac involvement: vegetations, valvular damage, and regurgitation.

Treatment
Patients with IE are hospitalized and given high-dose anti-microbial treatment to minimize cardiac damage. Despite treatment with current antibiotics, the fatality rate of IE remains between 20 and 70%.

Prevention
It should be emphasized that antibiotic prophylaxis does not preclude the development of IE in susceptible patients. It may minimize the risk. Dentists are encouraged to follow the current American Heart Association guidelines. See Tables 1–10, 1–11, & 1–12 on the next page.

ORAL HEALTH CONSIDERATIONS
The dentist is responsible for identifying patients at risk for IE. To accomplish this goal, the dentist should
- Obtain appropriate medical consultation when needed
- Identify dental procedures likely to cause bacteremia in susceptible patients

Table 1–10: Cardiac Conditions Associated with the Highest Risk of Adverse Outcome from Endocarditis for Which Prophylaxis with Dental Procedures is Reasonable

- Prosthetic cardiac valve or prosthetic material used for cardiac valve repair
- Previous infective endocarditis
- Congenital heart disease (CHD)*
- Unrepaired cyanotic congenital heart disease, including those with palliative shunts and conduits
- Completely repaired CHD with prosthetic material or device either by surgery or catheter intervention during the first 6 months after the procedure**
- Repaired CHD with residual defects at the site or adjacent to the site of a prosthetic patch or prosthetic device (which inhibit endothelialization)
- Cardiac transplantation recipients who develop cardiac valvulopathy

* Except for the conditions listed above, antibiotic prophylaxis is no longer recommended for any other form of CHD

** Prophylaxis is reasonable because endothelialization of prosthetic material occurs within 6 months after the procedure

Table 1–11: Dental Procedures for which Endocarditis Prophylaxis is Reasonable for Patients in Table 1–10

All dental procedures that involve manipulation of gingival tissue or the periapical region of teeth or perforation of the oral mucosa*

* The following procedures and events do not need prophylaxis: routine anesthetic injections through noninfected tissue, taking dental radiographs, placement of removable prosthodontic or orthodontic appliances, adjustment of orthodontic appliances, placement of orthodontic brackets, shedding of deciduous teeth and bleeding from trauma to the lips or oral mucosa.

Table 1–12: Regimens for a Dental Procedure

Situation	Agent	Regimen – Single Dose 30–60 minutes before procedure	
		Adults	Children
Oral	Amoxicillin	2 gm	50 mg/kg
Unable to take oral medication	Ampicillin OR Cefazolin OR ceftriaxone	2 g IM or IV 1 g IM or IV	50 mg/kg IM or IV 50 mg/kg IM or IV
Allergic to penicillins or ampicillin – oral	Cephalexin*† OR Clindamycin OR Azithromycin OR clarithromycin	2 g 600 mg 500 mg	50 m/kg 20 mg/kg 15 mg/kg
Allergic to penicillins or ampicillin and unable to take oral medication	Cefazolin OR ceftriaxone† OR Clindamycin phosphate	1 g IM or IV 600 mg IM or IV	50 mg/kg IM or IV 20 mg/kg IM or IV

IM = intramuscular; IV = intravenous.

* Or other first or second generation oral cephalosporin in equivalent adult or pediatric dosage.

† Cephalosporins should not be used in an individual with a history of anaphylaxis, angioedema, or urticaria with penicillins or ampicillin

- Select the appropriate antimicrobial regimen
- Eliminate all sources of infection that could serve as a nidus for cardiac infection

Additional Considerations for Preventing Endocarditis
- Optimal oral health should be encouraged.
- Oral irrigators and air abrasive polishing devices have been implicated in bacteremia, but the relationship to bacterial endocarditis is not known.
- Unanticipated bleeding may occur on some occasions. Institute antimicrobial prophylaxis within 2 hours following the procedure. Antibiotics administered more than 4 hours after the procedure probably have no effect.
- Edentulous patients may develop bacteremia from ulcers caused by ill-fitting dentures. Denture wearers should be encouraged to have periodic examinations or to return if discomfort develops. New dentures should be evaluated periodically to correct any problems that may cause mucosal ulceration.

The AAOM supports the recommendations of the American Heart Association on prevention of infective endocarditis.

CEREBROVASCULAR DISEASE

Definition

Strokes are a group of disorders involving sudden, focal interruption of cerebral blood flow that can result in neurologic deficit.

- Ischemic stroke (80%) results from thrombosis or embolism and is sometimes referred to as a "brain attack."
- Hemorrhagic stroke (20%) results from a vascular rupture producing a subarachnoid or intracerebral hemorrhage.

In Western countries, cerebral accidents are the fifth most common cause of death and the most common cause of neurologic disability.

Etiology

The occlusion of cerebral blood flow by emboli or thrombi can result in neurologic deficits.

- Anterior circulation stroke: unilateral symptoms
- Posterior circulation stroke: bilateral deficits that affect the level of consciousness

Chronology of Strokes

- Transient ischemic attack (TIA) is focal brain ischemia producing sudden neurologic deficits that last < 1 hour.
- TIAs are common in the middle-aged and elderly.
- The presence of TIAs increases the risk of a stroke.

- Stroke is suspected when there are sudden neurologic deficits consistent with brain damage.

Stroke Risk Factors

The risk factors listed in Table 1–13 may increase the likelihood of a patient suffering a stroke or TIA and/or significantly increase the risk for recurrent stroke or TIA.

Table 1–13: Risk Factors Associated with Stroke	
Non-modifiable Factors	**Modifiable Factors**

More prevalent if
 	
Age of patient:
 	
   • > 60 years of age
 	
Gender:
 	
   • males
 	
Race/ethnic group:
 	
   • African Americans
 	
Genetic factors:
 	
   • history of strokes
	Hypertension
	Hypercholesterolemia
	Diabetes mellitus
	Obesity
	Smoking
	Alcoholism
	Previous history of transient ischemic attacks
	   • Doubles risk for stroke
	Atrial fibrillation
	   • Fivefold increased risk
	Carotid artery stenosis
	Migraine headaches with aura
	Sedentary lifestyle

Table 1–14: Antiplatelet and Anticoagulant Medications Used In Patients with Cardiovascular Disease		
Medication	**Mode of Action**	**Laboratory Test**
Warfarin (Coumadin)	Vitamin K antagonist	INR
Aspirin	Inhibits platelet aggregation	Bleeding time*
Dipyridamole (Persantine)	Inhibits platelet aggregation	Bleeding time*
Aspirin/dipyridamole (Aggrenox)	Inhibits platelet aggregation	Bleeding time*
Ticlopidine (Ticlid)	Inhibits platelet aggregation	Bleeding time*
Clopidrogrel (Plavix)	Inhibits platelet aggregation	Bleeding time*
Dabigatran (Pradaxa)	Direct Thrombin Inhibitor	
Apixaban (Eliquis)		
Rivaroxaban (Xarelto)	Direct inhibitor factor Xa	
Betrixaban (Bevyxxa)		
Edoxaban (Savaysa)		
INR = international normalized ratio. *Bleeding time does not correlate well with clinical hemostasis unless > 20 minutes.		

ORAL HEALTH CONSIDERATIONS

- Obtain a comprehensive medical history.
- Identify the patient's medications: anticoagulant/antiplatelet medications.
- Determine and document the patient's INR (if taking an anticoagulant i.e., coumarin/warfarin).
- Identify the patient's risk factors for TIAs or stroke.
- Document and monitor the patient's blood pressure and pulse.
- Evaluate the patient's ability to perform effective oral hygiene activities, such as tooth brushing and flossing.
- Obtain profound anesthesia:
  - 2% Xylocaine with 1:100,000 epinephrine; no more than three carpules
  - NO retraction cord with epinephrine
- Minimize stress at the dental appointments: short appointments.

Minimal use of central nervous system depressants: opioid analgesic agents.

Table 1–15: Emergency Care for the Stroke Patient

If the dental patient demonstrates clinical signs and symptoms consistent with a transient ischemic attack or stroke, **IMMEDIATELY STOP THE DENTAL TREATMENT.**

- Activate the emergency medical system: Call 911 and document the time of the call.
- Be prepared to provide basic life support procedures.
- Place the patient in a comfortable position.
- Monitor the patient's vital signs.
- Provide oxygen to the patient.
- When emergency medical personnel arrive:
  - Provide them with information pertaining to the emergency
  - Medical history
  - Monitor Vital signs
  - Oxygen administration: time and flow rate
- Document the occurrence in the patient's dental record:
  - Time the emergency began
  - All dental office activities related to the emergency
  - Arrival time of emergency personnel
  - Emergency personnel medical procedures
  - Time of departure for the emergency room

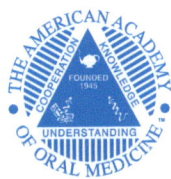

2 Allergic Reactions and Respiratory Disorders

ALLERGIC REACTIONS

Definition

Understanding allergies is critical because it enables the dentist to prepare for a medical emergency in the event of an allergic reaction. Dentists should also be able to recognize oral soft tissue changes occurring during allergic events. Modifications of treatment strategies may also be required if a patient is immunocompromised because of radiation, drug therapy, or an immune deficiency disorder. An apparently nonharmful substance (antigen) can trigger an immune response in certain individuals, and future exposures may lead to an inflammatory reaction. Allergic reactions can cause damage to affected tissues and even death in rare cases. Allergies result from an immune system reaction to an antigen (noninfectious foreign substance) owing to repetitive exposure. These immunologic hypersensitivity reactions are classified as follows:

Type I: Anaphylactic
- Involves immunoglobulin E (IgE) -mediated release of mediators such as histamine from mast cells
- Example: Asthma
- Response time: 1 to 30 minutes

Type II: Cytotoxic
- Involves IgG or IgM antibodies binding to cell surface antigens
- Usually, these antigens are endogenous, but they may be exogenous, such as that of drug-induced hemolytic anemia
- Example: Pemphigus
- Response time: Minutes to hours

Type III: Immune complex mediated
- Involves circulating antigens–antibody immune complexes deposits in small blood vessels
- Antigens may be endogenous or exogenous
- Example: Lupus erythematosus
- Response time: 3 to 8 hours

Type IV: Cell mediated (delayed)
- Mediated by T lymphocytes (not antibodies)
- Example: Tuberculosis testing and transplant rejection
- Response time: 48 to 72 hours

These reactions may be specific or nonspecific:
1. Nonspecific
   a. Mechanical reflexes such as coughing and sneezing
   b. Bactericidal secretions such as gastrointestinal acids and saliva enzymes
   c. Phagocyte action carried out by neutrophils and macrophages
   d. Circulating interferon and complement

2. Specific
   a. Humoral immunity: recognition and eradication of antigen mediated by B lymphocytes
   b. Cellular immunity: recognition and eradication of antigen mediated by T lymphocytes

It is beyond the scope of this summary to discuss the diagnosis and pathophysiology of each reaction. In summary, the humoral immune system reaction occurs immediately after contact with an antigen and may result in type I, II, and III hypersensitivity reactions. Type IV hypersensitivity reaction, on the other hand, involves the cellular immune system, and its onset is often delayed (Tables 2-1 and 2-2).

In the United States, 15 to 25% of the population is allergic to some substance, which includes 4.5% who have asthma, 4% who are allergic to insect stings, and 5% who are allergic to one or more drugs. There are approximately 500 deaths/year as a result of anaphylaxis. Allergic reactions tend to decrease with increasing age and have no genetic predilection. Allergies to multiple dental materials have been reported (Table 2-3).

Physical Evaluation/Status

Table 2–1: Clinical Manifestations of Allergic Response	
Type of Allergic Reaction	**Clinical Presentation**
I	Depends on the portal of entry of the allergen Examples: localized cutaneous swellings (hives), nasal or conjunctival discharge (allergic rhinitis and conjunctivitis), bronchial asthma, hay fever, or allergic gastroenteritis (food allergy). In the event of anaphylaxis, look for pruritus, flushing, urticaria, angioedema, rhinorrhea, wheezing, weakness, dizziness, dyspnea, and dysphagia In anaphylaxis, timing of treatment is critical as onset is usually sudden, rapidly progressing, and life-threatening
II	Necrosis Examples: transfusion reactions from mismatched blood type and rhesus incompatibility
III	Erythema, necrosis Examples: renal glomeruli and synovial membrane IV
IV	Erythema, induration Examples: graft-versus-host reaction, contact dermatitis, and drug hypersensitivity

Diagnosis

Table 2–2: Diagnostic Tests for Allergic Reactions	
Type of Allergic Reaction	**Diagnostic Test**
I	Skin testing Enzyme-linked immunoassay: measurement of total elevated IgE and specific IgE antibodies against allergens Association with antigen HLA-A2
II	Circulating antibodies in blood Presence of antibody and complement based on immunofluorescence study of reactive tissue
III	Presence of immunoglobulin and complement based on immunofluorescence study of reactive tissue

Medical Treatment

Treatment of anaphylaxis is time critical. Type I hypersensitivity treatment includes epinephrine, antihistamine, or corticosteroids. Type II and type III hypersensitivity reactions may be treated with anti-inflammatory or immunosuppressive agents.

Dental Management

In addition, patients on antihistamines for allergies may have xerostomia. Therefore, caution is advised with respect to prescribing cholinergic medications that could further dry the mouth. Caution is advised when prescribing erythromycin or ketoconazole if the patient is taking antihistamines, such as fexofenadine (Allegra), as this could result in increased plasma concentration of fexofenadine.

TABLE 2–3: Contact Dermatitis or Stomatitis to Dental Materials and Products
Dental amalgam (mercury)
Acrylic (free monomer, bench cured acrylic, uncured acrylic)
Composite resin
Nickel in Cr-Co prosthesis, gold restorations, and orthodontic wire
Impression material containing epimine
Eugenol
Rubber dam
Talcum powder
Toothpaste and mouthrinse

Management of a type I allergic reaction in the dental office demands knowledge and familiarity with emergency equipment and epinephrine delivery devices.

RESPIRATORY DISORDERS

ASTHMA

Definition

Asthma is a chronic inflammatory disease involving the airways. Current evidence supports a genetic predisposition. Asthma is characterized by hypertrophy of bronchial smooth muscle and obstruction of small airways by mucus. Symptoms include wheezing, breathlessness, and chest tightness. Symptoms may develop after exposure to allergens (pollens, house dust, tobacco smoke, animal dander), upper respiratory infections, stress, and exercise ("exercise-induced asthma"). Congestive heart failure may induce wheezing ("cardiac asthma"). Bronchial asthma affects about 8.4% of the US population—6.2 million children and 18.4 million adults. It is responsible for approximately 3,600 deaths per year in the United States. There are four types of asthma: extrinsic, intrinsic, exercise induced, and infectious. Each induces the release of histamine and cytokines that result in episodic bronchospasm associated with hypersecretion of mucus and decreased ciliary activity.

- *Extrinsic (allergic)*: Allergic stimulus, well-defined allergic history, elevated IgE levels (50–60%), positive skin tests, history of multiple family allergies (50% of cases), childhood or teenage onset, seasonal variations, and intermittent attacks.

- *Intrinsic (nonallergic)*: Nonallergic stimulus (idiopathic), no allergic history, low to normal IgE levels, normal skin tests, no significant history of family allergies, adult onset (over age 30 years), continuous asthmatic attacks, no seasonal changes, patient more prone to status asthmaticus.

- *Exercise induced*: Triggered by exercise and the inhalation of cold air. Children and young adults are more severely affected.

- *Infectious*: Develops as a result of viral or bacterial upper airway infections. Control is gained by effective antimicrobial treatment (bacterial) and supportive care (viral).

Physical Evaluation

Warning signs and symptoms include wheezing, chest tightness, a drop in forced expiratory volume (FEV), tachypnea, tachycardia, coughing, and dyspnea. **A severe asthmatic attack** is accompanied by diaphoresis and pulsus paradox (a decline of 10 mm Hg in blood pressure during inspiration compared with expiration or disappearance of the arterial pulse during slow respiration).

Status asthmaticus is an asthmatic attack that persists despite therapy and may last hours to days. Signs include fatigue, dehydration, hypoxia, peripheral vascular shock, and drug intoxication from attempted therapy. Diagnostic testing for asthma diagnosis includes chest radiographs, skin testing, histamine challenge test, sputum smears, blood counts (for eosinophilia), arterial blood gases (to rule out hypoxemia), enzyme-linked immunosorbent assay for allergen exposure, and spirometry (FEV).

Dental Management

The chief concerns from the standpoint of dental management are

- Avoidance of an asthmatic attack during the course of dental treatment that would create a medical emergency or compromise the result of the treatment
- Adequate preparedness to manage an asthmatic event should one occur

Evaluation

Assess patient risk status based on the medical classification scheme (Table 2-4) (e.g., frequency and severity of asthmatic attacks, type and amount of medications (Table 2-5), exercise tolerance, vital signs, current symptoms, nocturnal symptoms, and number and dates of most recent hospitalizations). Query the patient as to past triggers of attacks, being especially alert for medications, latex, surface disinfectants, and any history of attacks in dental or medical settings. Medical consultation with the patient's physician may be helpful in completing the history and assessing status.

Before Dental Care

1. Minimize stress by establishing rapport. Schedule short appointments whenever possible.
2. Remind patients to bring their medications and confirm that they have done so and that the medications are unexpired before starting treatment.
3. Review the patient's medications and be aware of potential drug interactions if administering or prescribing medications.
4. Sedation: If anxiolytic therapy is desired, N_2O–O_2 is generally the preferred choice. Short-acting benzodiazepines are acceptable. Barbiturates and opiates should be avoided because they have been prone to evoke asthmatic events in some patients.

TABLE 2–4: Medical Classification and Medical Management	
Classification	**Medical Management**
Mild intermittent Intermittent wheezing < 2 days/wk Exacerbations that are brief Asymptomatic between exacerbations Nocturnal symptoms < 2 days/mo FEV > 80% predicted	Daily medication not needed SA inhaled β_2-agonist (pirbuterol[Maxair]) as needed for symptom control Use more than 2 days/wk may indicate need for long-term control
Mild persistent Wheezing >2 d/wk (not daily) Exacerbations that affect activity and sleep Nocturnal asthma attacks 3-4 awakenings /mo Minor limitation with normal exercise Rare visits to emergency room (ER) FEV ≥ 80% predicted	Daily: inhaled anti-inflammatory, either corticosteroids, cromolyn, or nedocromil, sustained-release bronchodilator (theophylline or zafirlukast or zileuton) Symptom relief: short-acting inhaled β_2-agonist (pirbuterol [Maxair])
Moderate persistent Daily symptoms of wheezing (occur over several days) Daily use of SA β-agonist Exacerbation that affects activity and sleep and may last for days Nocturnal asthma attacks once/week More than minor limitation with normal exercise Rare ER visit FEV 60–80% predicted	Daily: inhaled corticosteroids with or without inhaled – β_2-agonist and/or bronchodilators (theophylline, zafirlukast, zileuton) Symptom relief: short-acting inhaled β_2-agonist (pirbuterol [Maxair])
Severe persistent Frequent/daily exacerbations Continual symptoms Frequent nocturnal asthma attacks (> 4 times/mo) Exercise intolerance FEV < 60% predicted Often results in hospital admission	Daily: inhaled corticosteroids (high dose) plus long-acting bronchodilator (β_2-agonist, theophylline) plus systemic (oral) corticosteroids. Symptom relief: SA inhaled β_2-agonist (pirbuterol [Maxair])
FEV = forced expiratory volume; SA = short acting.	

5. Moderate or severe persistent asthmatics: Medical consultation is advisable. Have the patient use an inhaler prophylactically prior to the appointment.

6. Severe persistent asthmatics: Medical consultation is strongly advised to assess the patient's risk for adverse events and determine appropriate treatment modifications. Consider sedation. Hospitalization should be considered for extensive procedures, multiple extractions, and advanced oral surgical procedures. Patients presenting with dental emergencies should be treated sufficiently to stabilize the urgent condition, with follow-up treatment postponed until any required medical consultation can be obtained and treatment modifications determined.

During Dental Care

Depending on the history of triggers, it may be advisable for particular patients to avoid or reduce the use of irritating odorants (such as certain surface disinfectants), rotary-derived particulate matter such as tooth enamel dust, methylmethacrylate, toothpaste, and foreign bodies, all of which have been documented to cause asthma attacks. For some patients, avoid cold operatory temperatures. For latex-sensitive patients, use nonlatex gloves and dental dams.

TABLE 2–5: Common Medications Used to Treat Asthma	
Bronchodilators	Long-acting β-agonists: salmeterol (Serevent), albuterol (Proventil, Repetabs, Volmax) extended release
	Short and intermediate acting: pirbuterol (Maxair), metaproterenol (Alupent, Metaprel), terbutaline (Bricanyl, Brethaire), isoetharine (Bronkometer, Bronkosol)
	Alpha and β-agonists: epinephrine (Primatene mist), methylxanthine
	Smooth muscle relaxant: theophylline (Theodur)
Anti-inflammatory agents	Corticosteroid inhalants: beclomethasone (Vancernase), budesonide (Pulmicort), flunisolide (Nasalide, AeroBid), fluticasone (Flonase, Flovent), triamcinolone (Azmacort)
	Corticosteroid/Beta 2 agonist: Breo Ellipta
	Leukotriene receptor inhibitors: zafirlukast (Accolate), montelukast (Singulair)
	Lipoxygenase pathway inhibitors: zileuton (Zyflo)
	Mast cell stabilizers: cromolyn (Intal), nedocromil (Tilade)
Anticholinergic	Ipratropium (Atrovent)

TABLE 2–6: Oral Manifestations Associated with Asthma		
Concern	*Diagnosis*	*Management*
Increased risk for caries from β-agonists that decrease salivary flow	Examine susceptible tooth surfaces, measure salivary flow	Frequent fluoride treatment; use prescription high-fluoride dentrifices
Increased risk for candidiasis from supplemental steroids in aerosols	Examine for oropharyngeal candidiasis	Antifungal agents, yogurt preparations, instruction on proper use of inhaler (rinse mouth after inhaler use)

The clinician should also be aware of the heightened risk of oral fungal infections and dental caries in these subjects (Table 2-6).

After Dental Care
Drug interactions: avoid macrolide antibiotics and clindamycin in patients who take theophylline because of increased risk of theophylline toxicity. Avoid use of aspirin, nonsteroidal anti-inflammatory drugs, and barbiturates as these are some of the drugs that most frequently elicit asthma attacks.

Managing Emergency (Asthma Attack) in the Dental Office
- Stop dental treatment, comfortably position the patient, and remove the rubber dam.
- Administer a β$_2$-agonist (e.g., albuterol, pirbuterol metered dose inhaler).
- Administer oxygen 2 to 3 L/min, by nasal canula, if available.
- Consider referral or transport for emergency medical care.

If the attack is refractory to the above attempts or the patient's condition deteriorates,

- Activate the emergency medical system (i.e., call "911," if available).
- Administer epinephrine 1:1,000/0.3 to 0.5 mL subcutaneously. If necessary, repeat doses may be administered as needed.
- If available, establish an IV line; administer 100 mg Solu-Cortef intravenously.
- Transfer the patient to an emergency room or urgent care facility.

CHRONIC OBSTRUCTIVE PULMONARY DISEASE
Definition
Chronic obstructive pulmonary disease (COPD) is characterized by airflow limitation that is not fully reversible. It is usually both slowly progressive and associated with an abnormal inflammatory response of the lungs to specific causes, such as noxious gases and particles. The term *COPD* encompasses chronic bronchitis and emphysema. Chronic bronchitis is characterized by the presence of chronic productive cough for at least 3 months during each of 2 consecutive years. It is necessary to exclude other causes of chronic cough, such as carcinoma of the lung, cystic fibrosis, *Mycobacterium tuberculosis* infection, chronic congestive heart failure, and bronchiectasis.

Emphysema is characterized by abnormal permanent enlargement of the respiratory bronchioles and alveoli accompanied by destruction of the alveolar septa without obvious fibrosis. By far the most important cause of COPD is cigarette (tobacco) smoking. It is estimated that cigarette smoking increases the risk of COPD 8.8-fold among males and 5.9-fold among females compared with nonsmokers. Other etiologies for COPD include cigar or pipe smoking, chronic occupational and environmental exposures such as inorganic dusts (coal, silica), grain or cotton dusts or acid fumes (sulfuric acid), and the absence of α_1-antitrypsin. In 2014 COPD was the third leading cause of death in the unitedStates. The prevalence of COPD in the United States is estimated to be 15.7 million people. COPD has a greater preponderance among males (14%) than females (8%). The incidence and prevalence of COPD increase with age and are highest among white males.

The pathogenesis of emphysema and the pathogenesis of chronic bronchitis are distinct. In emphysema, the loss of elastic recoil of the lungs occurs owing to enlargement of the air spaces distal to the terminal bronchioles and destruction of the alveolar walls. Therefore, obstruction during expiration (not inspiration) is caused by the collapse of unsupported and enlarged air spaces. The pathologic changes in chronic bronchitis are characterized by obstruction occurring with both inspiration and expiration, typically caused by small airway narrowing, mucous plugging, and peripheral airway collapse from loss of surfactant.

Physical Evaluation

The onset of COPD typically occurs in the fifth or sixth decade, years after exposure to the causative agent. Both chronic bronchitis and emphysema frequently occur together and share etiologic factors, making the distinction between the two diseases difficult. However, the signs and symptoms of one disease tend to predominate over the other, and this may be helpful in differentiating between the two entities (Table 2-7).

Diagnostic tests include pulmonary function tests, arterial blood gases, and sputum examination. Spirometry is the most important test for diagnosing and staging of COPD.

TABLE 2–7: Clinical Features of Chronic Bronchitis and Emphysema		
Feature	**Predominant Chronic Bronchitis (Blue Bloaters)**	**Predominant Emphysema (Pink Puffers)**
Age at onset (year)	~ 50	~ 60
Body morphology	Typically overweight	Typically thin, barrel cheated
Cough	Chronic productive	Not prominent
Sputum	Copious mucopurulent	Scant clear mucoid sputum
Respiration	Mild dyspnea No use of accessory muscles	Severe dyspnea Tachypnea, use of accessory muscles
Respiratory infections	Frequent	Infrequent
Cyanosis	Frequent (result of cor pulmonale)	Infrequent unless disease in late stage
Peripheral edema	Frequent (result of cor pulmonale)	Infrequent
PCO_2	Mild to severe hypercapnia	Normal
PO_2	Moderate to severe hypoxemia	Mild hypoxemia
Pulmonary function	Elastic recoil normal Obstruction on inspiration and expiration Lung capacity: normal to mild increased	Elastic recoil low Obstruction on expiration Lung capacity: moderate to severely
Chest radiograph	Increased thickness of bronchial walls Increased prominence of bronchovascular markings at the base of the lungs: "dirty chest" Cardiomegaly Diaphragms not flattened	Persistent and marked over distention of the lungs Flattened diaphragms Emphysematous bullae Small heart

Physical Status

COPD is classified into four stages according to the Global Initiative for Chronic Obstructive Lung Disease (GOLD):

1. Mild (FEV1 ≥ 80% predicted)
2. Moderate (50% ≤ FEV1 < 80% predicted)
3. Severe (30% ≤ FEV1 < 50% predicted)
4. Very Severe (FEV1 < 30% predicted)

Medical Treatment

Smoking cessation is the single most important factor in the management of COPD. Patients should also be encouraged to moderately exercise and eat a nutritious diet. Caution is advised in using medications that result in respiratory depression, such as sedatives and narcotics. Aggressive treatment of respiratory infections is vital, along with adjunctive physical therapy to mobilize lung secretions (Table 2-8).

Dental Management

BEFORE TREATMENT

1. Determine the basis for a COPD diagnosis, including onset, duration, and severity, associated symptoms such as dyspnea or orthopnea, current treatments, past surgical and nonsurgical treatments, and complications.

2. Review the entire medical history, paying close attention to cardiovascular issues such as hypertension and congestive heart failure (precautions specific to heart disease may be required).

3. Determine when the patient last visited the physician managing the COPD and the current results for dyspnea or orthopnea, spirometry, and blood gas test. Consider baseline complete blood count in severe bronchitis patients (consider medical consultation if the details are unclear).

4. Determine if COPD is exacerbated, including the presence of acute respiratory infections or continued smoking.

5. Check pulse and blood pressure: tachycardia, irregular rhythm, and elevated blood pressure may suggest toxic reactions to sympathomimetic agents, anticholinergic agents, bronchodilators, or methylxanthines.

6. Consider performing dental treatment in a hospital setting in anticipation of medical complications for stage IIB and stage III COPD

| TABLE 2–8: Medical Management of COPD ||
Intervention	*Indication*
Oxygen	• Nocturnal or ambulatory continuous low-flow oxygen • Severe COPD • During exacerbations • Patients must be hypoxemic • Avoid hypercapnia with high-flow oxygen therapy
Antibiotics	• For respiratory infections • Consider azithromycin, levofloxacin, amoxicillin-clavunate, and cefuroxime
Bronchodilators	• Used for chronic bronchitis • Anticholinergic: ipratropium bromide • Sympathomimetic: albuterol or metaproterenol
Methylxanthines	• For sleep-related respiratory disturbances • Failed bronchodilator therapy • Theophylline
Corticosteroids	• Chronic bronchitis (increase eosinophilia presence) • Prednisone
Surgical	• Bullectomy • Reduction pneumoplasty • Lung transplantation

DURING TREATMENT

1. If orthopnea is present, place the patient in a semisupine position to avoid respiratory distress.

2. Consider the use of a pulse oximeter to determine SpO_2. An oxygen saturation of < 90% warrants immediate termination of dental treatment and referral to a physician.

3. Local anesthetic with a vasoconstrictor is not contraindicated, but dose limitation may be required if the patient has tachycardia or hypertension.

4. Avoid use of a rubber dam in severely compromised patients.

5. Consider use of low-flow O_2 (2 L/min) via a nasal cannula.

6. NO_2 use is contraindicated in patients with severe COPD or emphysema.

7. Avoid use of medications that can cause respiratory depression, such as narcotics and barbiturates.

8. Low-dose benzodiazepines may be used with caution if sedation is required. Preoperative respiratory function should be assessed by a physician.

9. Assess the presence of adrenal suppression and insufficiency in patients using corticosteroids.

AFTER TREATMENT

1. Avoid the use of erythromycin if the patient is taking methylxanthine (theophylline) as this may result in inhibition of cytochrome P-450 and elevation of methylxanthine levels.

2. Take caution with the use of postoperative narcotics in labile patients.

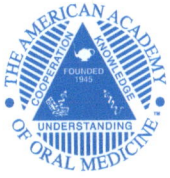

3 Metabolic Diseases

DIABETES MELLITUS

Description

Diabetes mellitus (DM) is a chronic illness consisting of a group of metabolic disorders of multiple etiologies characterized by hyperglycemia resulting from defects in insulin secretion, insulin action, or both, which gives rise to disturbances of carbohydrate, protein and lipid metabolism.

Epidemiology

An estimated 29.1 million Americans, or 9.3% of the US population, have DM. Approximately 1.4 million new cases are diagnosed each year. It is the seventh underlying cause of death in the United States.

Pathogenesis

The chronic hyperglycemia of diabetes is associated with long-term damage, dysfunction, and failure of various organs, especially the eyes, kidneys, nerves, heart, and blood vessels. Cardiovascular disease is a major contributor to morbidity for individuals with diabetes and the major cause of mortality.

Table 3–1: Classification and Key Features of Diabetes Mellitus	
Classification	**Key Features**
Type 1	• Accounts for 5–10% of cases of DM • Very little insulin secretion, usually leading to absolute insulin deficiency • Primarily owing to autoimmune destruction of pancreatic beta cells but may also be idiopathic • Multiple genetic and ill-defined environmental etiologic factors; obesity not paramount • Peak incidence is childhood and adolescence but can occur at any age • Children and adolescents may initially present with ketoacidosis, unexplained weight loss
Type 2	• Accounts for 90–95% of cases of DM • A progressive defect of insulin secretion on the background of insulin resistance • Multifactorial, poorly defined etiology; risk factors include genetic predisposition, increasing age (> 45 years), sedentary lifestyle, hypertension, dyslipidemia • Obesity is paramount, fueling insulin resistance • High-risk ethnic groups include African Americans, Latinos, and Native Americans • Classic symptoms (polyuria, polydipsia) may be absent owing to gradual onset of hyperglycemia
Other specific types	• Relatively uncommon • Usually secondary to genetic defects in beta cell function or insulin action, pancreatic disease or infection, chemical or drug therapy (transplant or HIV therapy), toxins, rare genetic syndromes
Gestational DM	• Complicates from 4.6–9.2% of pregnancies; the higher percentages in African Americans, Latinos, Native Americans, the obese, and those who have a strong family history of DM • Glucose intolerance with onset of pregnancy often resulting in large infants at birth.
DM = diabetes mellitus; HIV = human immunodeficiency virus	

TABLE 3−2: Diagnosis
Polyuria, polydipsia, and unexplained weight loss plus casual plasma glucose concentration ≥ 200 mg/dL (11.1 mmol/L). Casual is defined as any time of day without regard to time since last meal.
OR
Fasting plasma glucose ≥ 126 mg/dL (7.0 mmol/L). Fasting is defined as no caloric intake for at least 8 h.
OR
2-hour plasma glucose ≥ 200 mg/dL (11.1 mmol/L) during an oral glucose tolerance test. This test is not recommended for routine clinical use.   *OR*   Glycosylated Hemoglobin (HbA1c) ≥ 6.5%

TABLE 3−3: Physical Signs and the Importance of Severity of Symptoms
Systemic complications of diabetes mellitus resulting from chronic hyperglycemia may include
• Cardiovascular disease = the major cause of mortality with diabetes   • Nephropathy = early recognition important to slow progression and injury   • Retinopathy = the most frequent cause of new cases of adult blindness   • Peripheral arterial disease = specific inquiry about foot care is very important   • Susceptibility to infection = decreased sensitivity, impaired skin blood flow   • Impaired wound healing = wound care may require special management

Laboratory Interpretation

- Normal fasting plasma glucose = < 100 mg/dL (5.6 mmol/L)
- Impaired fasting glucose (IFG) = 100 to 125 mg/dL (5.6–6.9 mmol/L)
- Abnormal or provisional diabetes to be confirmed = ≥ 126 mg/dL (7.0 mmol/L)

Patients with IFG are referred to as having "prediabetes," indicating the relatively high risk for the development of diabetes. The oral glucose tolerance test is rarely performed in the initial screening of clinical practice but may be of value when used by the physician to evaluate a referred provisional diabetic.

Glycosylated Hemoglobin (HbA1c)

Glycosylation is a non-enzymatic addition of glucose to hemoglobin. The glycated hemoglobin assay (HbA1c, often called A1C) measures the percentage of glycosylated hemoglobin on circulating red blood cells and reflects the plasma glucose level over the preceding 2-3 months. Higher plasma glucose levels over time correspond to greater levels of HbA1c. It is used for definitive diagnosis of DM, for monitoring the progress of the disease and it is a predictor for the development of chronic complications in diabetes. In general, the target for diabetic patients is to have the HbA1c at ≤ 7%.

MEDICAL MANAGEMENT

The objective of medical management of DM is to maintain tight glycemic control, which inhibits the onset and delays the progression of complications of diabetes. Essential components of disease management include appropriate pharmacologic regimens (oral hypoglycemic agents and parenteral agents including insulin), comprehensive education in self-management, (including diet control, exercise, and frequent self monitoring of blood glucose) as well as prevention and treatment of chronic complications of diabetes.

Oral Hypoglycemics

Prior to 1995, there was only one type of oral medication used to treat diabetes. Many oral agents now exist, including those with a dry powder formulation for inhalation use with type 1 or 2 diabetes. An extensive list of specific medications used to treat diabetes is beyond the scope of this monograph. However, the clinician should be aware of the major oral agents and their mechanism of action as listed in Table 3-5.

PARENTERAL AGENTS

Insulin

All type 1 and some type 2 diabetics use exogenous insulin. Inhaled insulin, a dry powder formulation of rapid-acting human insulin, is also being used with type 1 or 2 diabetes. There are numerous insulin preparations classified by onset, peak, and duration of activity that vary with the individual product (Table 3-6).

More recently, other parenteral agents such as synthetic analogues of human amylin as well as glucagonlike peptide-1 (GLP-1) analogues are available for self-administration to supplement insulin at mealtime. Dipeptidyl peptidase-4 inhibitor (gliptins) have shown a promising effectiveness and safety in reducing HbA1c in type 2 diabetes mellitus.

TABLE 3–4: Signs and Symptoms of Inadequate Glycemic Control		
Inadequate Glycemic Control	Hypoglycemia	Hyperglycemia
Onset	Rapid (min–h)	Prolonged
Precipitating factors	Excessive insulin level Excessive sulfonylurea Medications Weight loss Increased physical activity Inadequate carbohydrate	Inadequate insulin level Weight gain (obesity) Lack of physical activity Pregnancy Hyperthyroidism Glucocorticosteroids Acute infection, stress fever
Clinical manifestations	Diminished cerebral function Mood changes Lethargy Hunger Sweating Tachycardia Anxiety, agitation Bizarre behavior	Polydipsia Polyphagia Polyuria Weight loss Acetone/fruity breath odor Dehydration Tachycardia Hypotension Hyperventilation/Kussmaul respirations
Adverse sequelae	Unconsciousness Seizures Hypotension Hypothermia	Ketoacidosis Coma

TABLE 3–5: Oral Hypoglycemics	
Drug	Action
Sulfonylureas	Increases insulin secretion
Meglitinides and phenylalanine derivatives	Increases insulin secretion
Alpha-glucosidase inhibitors	Decrease carbohydrate absorption, preventing a rise in glucose after meals
Biguanides	Reduce hepatic glucose production; requires the presence of insulin
Thiazolinediones	Decrease glucose by increasing muscle and liver use of insulin; requires the presence of insulin
DPP–4 inhibitors	Increase and prolong activity of incretin hormone, which increases insulin synthesis and release
Sodium/glucose cotransporter 2 inhibitors	Increases urinary glucose excretion
Combination drugs	Combination of two medications from a different chemical class, each retaining its effect, acting complementarily

ORAL HEALTH CARE CONSIDERATIONS/ DENTAL MANAGEMENT

Oral Manifestations

Uncontrolled or poorly controlled diabetes is associated with increased susceptibility to oral infections, including periodontitis. Diminished salivary flow and increased glucose concentration in oral fluids and tissues may alter plaque microflora and contribute to the development of periodontal disease, dental caries, and oral candidiasis.

Periodontal diseases may be more severe in diabetics with more advanced systemic complications, and impaired

TABLE 3–6: Insulin Preparations for Injection			
Type	*Onset of Activity*	*Peak Activity (h)*	*Effective Duration (h)*
Rapid acting	10 – 30 min	0.5 – 3	3 – 5
Intermediate acting	10 – 30 min	2.4	Up to 24
Short acting	30 – 60 min	2 – 5	5 – 8
Intermediate short	30 – 60 min	0.5 – 12	Up to 24
Intermediate	1 – 2 h	2 – 12	14 – 24
Long acting	1.5 h	None	20 – 24

wound healing can be observed. Periodontal infection and treatment also may have the potential to alter glycemic control. Oral burning and taste disturbances are also common in patients with DM.

Since prevention plays a primary role in the control of periodontal disease, patients with diabetes may require more frequent plaque removal and scaling. Smoking increases the risk of periodontal disease, and tobacco cessation should be an integral component of dental treatment.

Prior to Dental Care

- Medical history should include disease severity, degree of control, specific medication/regimens, dose and times of administration, compliance with medication and diet, and track record for infections.
- Consult the patient's physician if control is inadequate or the dental treatment plan will necessitate adjustment of a normal diet or medication regimen.
- Morning, short appointments are generally preferable and should not extend into normal meal or snack times.
- Ensure that the patient has maintained normal dietary intake and medication regimen prior to appointments.
- If inadequate glycemic control is suspected, check blood glucose level with commercially available monitor prior to initiating treatment; administer oral carbohydrate or defer treatment as necessary.
- HbA1C test results should be assessed when infection is present or extensive surgical procedures are planned.

During Dental Care

- Hypoglycemia requires termination of treatment and administration of approximately 15 g of a fast-acting carbohydrate (i.e., fruit juice, sugar, or candy) to the conscious patient.
- Loss of consciousness with suspected hypoglycemia requires immediate medical assistance; provide basic life support and administer IV dextrose (50%) or IM glucagons (1 mg) if possible.
- Hyperglycemia is rare and requires medical intervention and insulin administration.
- If the diagnosis is uncertain and signs or symptoms are mistaken for hypoglycemia, it is generally safe to administer a small amount of glucose without adverse effects.

After Dental Care

- Infection risk assessment: Postoperative antibiotic coverage may be necessary for patients with poor glycemic control who have significant oral infections or who have undergone extensive surgical procedures.
- Postoperative analgesics: Salicylates increase insulin secretion and may potentiate the action of sulfonylurea drugs, resulting in altered glycemic control. Therefore, aspirin and aspirin-containing compounds should be avoided.

ADRENAL GLAND DISORDERS

Definition

Adrenal gland disorders are abnormalities that result in the overproduction or underproduction of secretory products (hormones) of the adrenal gland(s). The adrenal glands are responsible for producing the adrenal steroids, mineralocorticoids, and norepinephrine.

Etiology

Clinically, adrenal disease can be related to primary endocrinopathies as well as autoimmune, infectious, neoplastic, or iatrogenically induced disorders. Overproduction is often due to tumors, whereas underproduction is often the result of destruction of the adrenal cortex of one or both glands. Excessive production of glucocorticoids is known as **Cushing disease**. Primary adrenal insufficiency is known as **Addison disease**.

Glucocorticoid Deficiency

Glucocorticoid deficiency disorders are generally divided into two categories:

- Primary adrenal insufficiency results from progressive destruction of the adrenal glands. Causes include tuberculosis and other chronic granulomatous diseases, autoimmune disorders, and neoplasms.
- Secondary adrenal insufficiency results from hypothalamic-pituitary disease and suppression by chronic exogenous steroid administration.

Epidemiology

The incidence of Addison disease (endogenous glucocorticoid deficiency) is estimated between 40 – 60 cases per 1 million population. It is equally distributed in both sexes and among all age groups. Noniatrogenic causes of glucocorticoid excess (Cushing syndrome) are relatively rare.

Clinical Features

The clinical features of Addison's disease do not usually appear until at least 90% of the glandular tissue has been destroyed.

TABLE 3–7: Signs and Symptoms of Glucocorticoid Insufficiency
• Weakness, fatigability
• Weight loss
• Hypotension
• Gastrointestinal dysfunction (anorexia, nausea, vomiting, diarrhea, abdominal pain)
• Melanin-based hyperpigmentation of the skin and mucous membranes

Acute adrenal insufficiency is a rare but potentially life-threatening situation. Signs and symptoms include rapidly evolving agitation, confusion, fever, abdominal pain, and a drop in blood pressure.

Glucocorticoid Excess (Cushing Syndrome)

Cushing syndrome is due to increased production of cortisol by the adrenal glands. Etiologies include adrenocorticotropic hormone (ACTH)-dependent causes, including pituitary adenoma (Cushing disease), ectopic ACTH-secreting neoplasms (e.g., carcinoma or small cell lung carcinoma), ACTH-independent causes (e.g., adrenal adenoma), and exogenous iatrogenic causes (e.g., prolonged use of glucocorticoids).

Physical Evaluation

TABLE 3–8: Signs and Symptoms of Cushing Syndrome Related to the Actions of Glucocorticoids
• Increased body weight and abnormal adipose deposition (truncal obesity, moon face, buffalo hump)
• Violaceous cutaneous striae and easy bruising
• Hirsutism
• Acne
• Proximal muscle weakness and fatigability
• Headache
• Hypertension
• Emotional changes (irritability, emotional lability, depression)
• Menstrual dysfunction
• Osteopenia, osteoporosis, Insulin resistance, impaired glucose tolerance

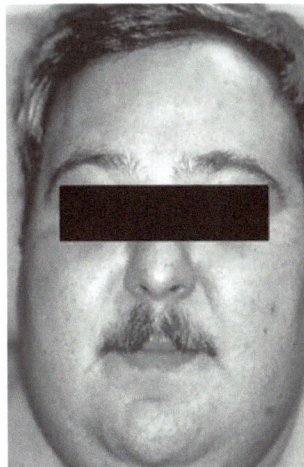

FIGURE 3-1: *Moon-shaped face in a patient who has Cushing syndrome*

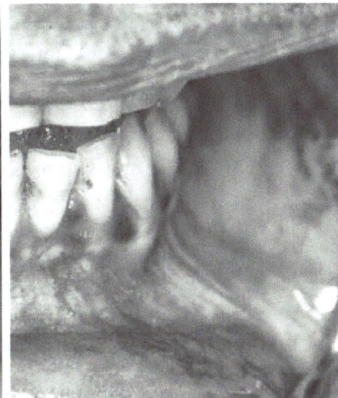

FIGURE 3-2: *Melanin deposition in the buccal mucosa and tongue in a patient with Addison disease.*

MEDICAL MANAGEMENT

Cushing disease is usually surgically managed by excision of the pituitary tumor causing the abnormality. The treatment of choice for **Addison disease** is daily hormone replacement with a corticosteroid (hydrocortisone, prednisone, or dexamethasone) and a mineralocorticoid (fludrocortisone [Florinef]).

DENTAL MANAGEMENT

- Patients with either primary adrenal insufficiency or those on chronic exogenous steroids may be unable to increase endogenous steroid production to respond appropriately to the stress of invasive or extensive dental procedures. Routine dental procedures can be performed without modifications.

- Dentists should be aware of precipitating factors including significant adrenal insufficiency, poor health status, infection and painful invasive procedures.
- Acute adrenal insufficiency (adrenal crisis), although rare, is more likely during the postoperative period, when pain and hypovolemia may be developing.
- Features include weakness, fatigue, and hypotension.
- If untreated, the condition can evolve into shock, coma, and death. Life support measures, including administration of glucocorticosteroid (100 mg hydrocortisone IM or IV), are indicated.

Patients should be assessed on an individual basis and consultation with the patient's physician is recommended to determine the extent of adrenal suppression and the need for steroid supplementation (Table 3-9).

TABLE 3–9: Steroid Supplementation Guidelines
• Patient has a previous history of regular steroid use that was discontinued recently or in the past or is currently using topical or inhalation steroids: **no supplementation is required for routine dental procedures**.
• Patient is currently taking steroids and routine dental procedures are planned: **no supplementation is required for routine dental procedures**.
• Patient is currently taking steroids and minor to moderate surgery is being performed: Ensure that patient takes 25 to 75 mg of hydrocortisone equivalent prior to procedure and ensure effective local anesthesia and adequate postoperative pain control. **Monitor blood pressure throughout procedure**.
• Patient is currently taking steroids (or has low adrenal reserve) and major surgery (lasting more than 1 h) or significant blood loss is anticipated: **The glucocorticoid target is about 100 to 150 mg/d of hydrocortisone equivalent for the day of surgery and at least 1 postoperative day. Ensure effective local anesthesia and adequate postoperative pain control. Monitor blood pressure throughout procedure and postoperative period**.

Prescribing Steroids

Because of the potential profound and varied metabolic effects of steroids, care must be taken in their administration. Prolonged systemic steroid therapy (> 1 month) may exacerbate many systemic conditions, including, but not limited to, hypertension, diabetes mellitus, and osteoporosis. Gastrointestinal ulcers, cataracts, secondary infections, and possible reactivation of dormant microbes (e.g., herpes, Mycobacterium tuberculosis) may follow prolonged steroid therapy. Common initial complaints include urinary frequency, excess appetite, sleeplessness, and agitation.

Most adverse reactions to corticosteroids occur after 2-weeks of usage. If systemic steroids are prescribed by the dentist, the general rule is to prescribe a higher dose for a short period of time (burst therapy) whenever possible rather than a lower dose over a protracted period of time. Topical steroid therapy for oral mucosal disorders has been reported to be safe for short-term therapy.

THYROID DISORDERS
Description
Definition
Thyroid gland dysfunction can result in either decreased or excessive production of thyroid hormone.

Epidemiology
Thyroid disorders are generally more common in females than in males. In the United States population, the prevalence of hypothyroidism is estimated at 4.6% while in iodine-deficient areas of the world, the incidence of this disease is 10 to 20 times higher.

The prevalence of hyperthyroidism in females is 100 per 100,000 and 33 per 100,000 in males. The usual age at onset is between 20 and 40 years.

Pathogenesis
Abnormalities in the anterior pituitary or the thyroid gland itself can result in abnormal thyroid hormone production.

HYPOTHYROIDISM
Hypothyroidism results from decreased secretion of thyroid hormone from the thyroid gland. The disease is classified into primary and secondary diseases. Primary disease is characterized by failure of the thyroid gland to produce triiodothyronine (T3) and thyroxine (T4) hormones. The most common causes of primary hypothyroidism include autoimmune and post-ablative (iatrogenic) damage to the thyroid gland. In secondary disease, the thyroid gland is

TABLE 3-10: Relative Potencies of Glucocorticoids			
Systemic Equivalent Doses for Glucocorticoids		Relative Topical Agent Potencies	
United States Pharmacopeia Name	mg		
		Ultra potent	Clobetasol propionate 0.05% Halobetasol propionate 0.05%
Dexamethasone Triamcinolone Methylprednisolone Prednisone Cortisone Hydrocortisone	0.75 4.0 4.0 5.0 25.0 20.0	Potent	Fluocinonide 0.05% Desoximetasone 0.25%
		Moderately potent	Triamcinolone acetonide0.5%, 0.1% Betamethasone dipropionate0.05% Betamethasone valerate 0.1%
		Mildly potent	Hydrocortisone 1.0%, 0.5%

normal; however, either the pituitary gland fails to secrete adequate thyroid-stimulating hormone (TSH) or the hypothalamus fails to secrete thyrotropin-releasing hormone.

HYPERTHYROIDISM

The most common cause of hyperthyroidism in the United States is **Graves's disease.** This is an autoimmune condition in which thyroid-stimulating immunoglobulin binds to and activates TSH receptors in the thyroid, increasing

hormone synthesis and release, resulting in a diffusely enlarged thyroid gland.

Physical Evaluation

The signs and symptoms of thyroid disorders are related to the rapidity of onset, duration, and severity of illness; extent of hormone imbalance; and age of the patient (Table 3-13). A thyroid radioactive iodine (I-123) imaging study may be completed in suspected cases of hyperthyroidism.

TABLE 3-11: Causes of Hypothyroidism
Chronic autoimmune thyroiditis (Hashimoto thyroiditis) Surgical removal of the thyroid gland Radioactive iodine therapy External irradiation Drug induced (e.g., lithium, sulfonamides) Pituitary and hypothalamic disease

TABLE 3-12: Causes of Hyperthyroidism
Toxic adenoma Toxic multinodular goiter Painful subacute thyroiditis Silent thyroiditis, including lymphocytic and postpartum variations Iodine-induced hyperthyroidism Excessive pituitary thyroid-stimulating hormone

TABLE 3-13: Signs and Symptoms of Thyroid Disorders		
Tissue	Hypothyroidism	Hyperthyroidism
Central nervous system	Ataxia; mental slowness; dementia; forgetfulness; decreased concentration	Insomnia; tremors; sleep disturbances; nervousness; irritability; agitation; emotional lability
Skin	Dry, rough skin; coarse hair; nonpitting edema(myxedema)	Warm, moist, smooth skin; fine, thin hair; onchyolysis; excessive perspiration
Metabolic	Weight gain; cold intolerance; decreased basal metabolic rate	Weight loss; heat intolerance; increased appetite
Cardiovascular	Bradycardia; hypertension; pericardial effusion; anemia	Palpitations; atrial fibrillation; tachycardia
Respiratory	Depressed ventilatory drive	Dyspnea
Gastrointestinal	Hypomotility; constipation	Hypermotility; hyperdefecation; diarrhea

Laboratory Test	Hypothyroidism	Hyperthyroidism
Thyroid function tests	Decreased free T_4 33% have decreased free T_3	Increased serum and free T_3/T_4
TSH	Elevated serum TSH	Decreased serum TSH
Thyroid autoantibodies	Elevated antithyroglobulin	Elevated antithyroperoxidase

TABLE 3–14: Laboratory Studies

T_3 = triiodothyronine; T_4 = thyroxine; TSH = thyroid-stimulating hormone.

High uptake of I-123 are evident in patients with Graves's disease and toxic nodular goiter, whereas low uptake of I-123 would be seen in patients with subacute thyroiditis.

Medical Treatment

Hypothyroidism

The primary goal is to restore and maintain normal thyroid function. Replacement of T_4 is the treatment of choice, and levothyroxine is the medication most commonly used for this purpose. Starting dose is usually 25 to 50 μg per day and is titrated according to the individual's response. Patients generally take levothyroxine indefinitely and must be assessed periodically for possible dosage adjustments.

Hyperthyroidism

Treatment of hyperthyroidism may consist of medication, radioactive iodine therapy, or surgery. Antithyroid medications, such as methimazole and propylthiouracil, inhibit the synthesis of thyroid hormones and may be effective in treating this disease. However, a high rate of recurrent hyperthyroidism (approximately 50%) has been reported after a year or more of therapy. Radioactive iodine 131 (I-131) is another treatment modality in which the compound is taken up by the thyroid gland and destroys thyroid follicular cells. There is a high incidence of hypothyroidism following radioactive I-131 therapy, and permanent, postablative hypothyroidism occurs in approximately 33% of patients receiving this treatment. Surgical options include subtotal removal of the thyroid gland, which may result in hypothyroidism. Patients who develop hypothyroidism from either of the above treatment modalities would require lifelong hormone replacement therapy.

Physical Status

Hypothyroidism

Hypothyroidism causes a slowing of metabolic processes, and when it occurs in utero or shortly after birth, the syndrome is termed **cretinism** and is characterized by abnormalities in intellectual and physical development. In adults, hypothyroidism is manifested as **myxedema** and is characterized by widespread slowing of metabolic processes, formation of nonpitting edema, and diminished cardiac output. Myxedema coma is a rare but life-threatening emergency; it occurs most frequently in hypothyroid patients with severe myxedema (either spontaneously or as a result of cold exposure), intake of medications (such as analgesics and sedatives), or infection. Clinical signs are severe hypothermia, hypoventilation, hypoxia, and hypotension.

If treated early, hypothyroidism generally carries a good prognosis. If compliance with medication is poor or if treatment is interrupted, relapse will occur. If hypothyroidism is left untreated, it may progress to myxedema and coma.

Hyperthyroidism

The most common cause of hyperthyroidism is Graves's disease, and patients with this condition have specific clinical manifestations resulting from the underlying autoimmune nature of the disease. Exophthalmos is a classic feature of this disease and is characterized by protrusion of the globe of the eye, proptosis, and restriction of eye movement. This is caused by edema of retro-orbital connective tissue and extraocular muscles; keratitis and corneal ulceration may ensue.

Thyrotoxic crisis (thyroid storm) is a life-threatening condition that occurs most frequently in patients with severe thyrotoxicosis. It is usually precipitated by systemic illness, emotional stress, surgery, and/or infection. Clinical signs and symptoms include fever, restlessness, tachycardia, atrial fibrillation, pulmonary edema, tremor, sweating, stupor, and progression to coma and death if treatment is not provided.

Hyperthyroidism generally has a good prognosis with most etiologies when appropriately diagnosed and treated. Thyrotoxic crisis is the major complication of the disease and is associated with high morbidity and mortality if untreated.

DENTAL MANAGEMENT

Assessment of the thyroid gland should be an integral component of the head and neck examination. Visualization of the thyroid gland requires observation of the contour of the neck from the side while the patient swallows. Palpation of the thyroid is performed by standing behind the patient, using the fingers of both hands to identify the isthmus located just below the cricoid cartilage. While exerting gentle pressure, the patient should be asked to take small sips of water and swallow; as the gland is palpated, it will move superiorly when the patient swallows. Thyroid enlargements and irregularities such as nodules can be identified via this examination technique. In addition, the posterior dorsal tongue should be examined for a nodule that could represent ectopic lingual thyroid tissue.

A thorough history and physical assessment are required for all patients with thyroid disease.

Hypothyroidism

A specific diagnosis of hypothyroidism should be established, and the patient's current medications (name, dosage) should be documented in the dental chart. The patient's current clinical disease status and stability must be assessed prior to initiation of dental treatment. If the clinician suspects poorly controlled disease, consultation with the patient's physician regarding disease status is recommended and recent thyroid function tests (within the past 6 to 12 months) should be evaluated prior to initiation of dental treatment. Patients with well-controlled hypothyroidism require no special precautions for routine or emergent dental treatment in the absence of other concurrent medical problems. For patients with undiagnosed, untreated, or poorly controlled hypothyroidism, elective dental care should be deferred until the disease is controlled and the patient reestablishes proper thyroid function.

Hyperthyroidism

The same treatment guidelines apply to patients with hyperthyroidism. Patients with well-controlled disease require no special precautions for routine or emergent dental treatment in the absence of other concurrent medical problems. The use of epinephrine or other pressor amines must be avoided in untreated or poorly controlled hyperthyroidism as it can exacerbate symptoms of tachycardia, dyspnea, and fatigue. Patients with well-controlled disease may be given normal concentrations of these vasoconstrictors. Patients with undiagnosed, untreated, or poorly controlled hyperthyroidism are at increased risk for development of thyrotoxic crisis (thyroid storm), and this condition may be precipitated by stress, acute oral infection,

or vigorous thyroid gland palpation. The clinician should take appropriate measures to reduce stress, prevent and/or treat acute oral infection, and avoid vigorous palpation of the thyroid gland to avert precipitating this life-threatening condition. The emergency management for a hyperthyroid crisis is presented in Table 3-15.

TABLE 3–15: Emergency Management for a Hyperthyroid Crisis
If the patient goes into a hyperthyroid crisis, terminate the dental procedure, begin emergency therapy as described, and obtain immediate medical assistance:
• Cool the patient with cold towels or ice packs
• Administer hydrocortisone (100–300 mg, IM or IV)
• Monitor the patient's vital signs
• Be prepared to initiate cardiopulmonary resuscitation

Although it is rare, patients using methimazole or propylthiouracil may be at increased risk for development of agranulocytosis; this may be evaluated via a complete blood count with differential. Oral findings associated with hyperthyroidism may include more aggressive periodontal disease, increased susceptibility to caries, osteoporosis of the maxilla and/or mandible, and accelerated dental eruption in children and adolescents. Patients medically treated with radioactive iodine 131 may experience salivary hypofunction, ductal blockage and swelling.

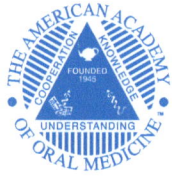

4   Gastrointestinal, Liver and Renal Diseases

INFLAMMATORY BOWEL DISEASE

Definition

There are numerous diseases of the gastrointestinal tract. In this guide, the focus is inflammatory bowel disease (IBD). IBD is composed of two painful and destructive chronic disorders: **Crohn disease** and **ulcerative colitis**. Crohn's disease is an inflammatory disease of the entire wall of the bowel that produces "skip" ulcerations along any point of the digestive tract from the mouth to the anus. It most commonly involves the terminal ileum. Ulcerative colitis is an inflammatory mucosal disease limited in scope to the large intestine and rectum. Although the cause of IBD is unknown, genetic (i.e., the *Nod2/Card15* gene) and microbial factors appear to alter innate immune responses that lead to features of the disease.

Epidemiology

Ten new cases of IBD per 100,000 persons are diagnosed annually in the United States and Europe, and approximately 1 million persons in the United States live with the disease. IBD appears primarily in young adulthood (20–40 years of age). Ulcerative colitis occurs equally in men and women. There is a slight predilection for women with Crohn disease. First-degree relatives of IBD patients are 10 times more likely to develop the condition.

Pathogenesis

Crohn disease is a chronic and relapsing disease characterized by elevated levels of cytokines and noncaseating granulomas that produce segmental intestinal ulcers (skip lesions) that are intervened by normal mucosa. Affected sites most often are the distal ileum, proximal colon, and rectum. Repeated inflammatory attacks lead to a thickened bowel wall, irregular glandular openings, fissures, erosions, strictures and nodular or "cobblestoned" mucosa. Long-standing disease increases the risk for colorectal cancer.

Ulcerative colitis produces epithelial erosions in the colon-rectum region that may spread to involve the entire large intestine and the ileum. The disease is persistent and characterized by exacerbations of edema, hemorrhage, abscesses, and submucosal fibrosis. Clinical attacks are followed by periods of remissions. Repeated fibrosis leads

TABLE 4–1: Signs and Symptoms of Inflammatory Bowel Disease		
Tissue	**Crohn Disease**	**Ulcerative Colitis**
Main gastrointestinal features	Symptoms vary from patient to patient according to site of involvement Typical features: recurrent or persistent diarrhea (often without blood), abdominal cramps (colicky pain, aggravated by eating), anorexia, weight loss, unexplained fever, malaise	Attacks of diarrhea, rectal bleeding (or bloody diarrhea), and abdominal cramps
Complications	Intestinal fissuring, fistulae, and abscess formation that lead to malabsorption, weight loss, growth failure, anemia, osteoporosis	Dehydration, fatigue, weight loss, fever, malabsorption, growth failure
Extraintestinal manifestations	Arthritis, erythema nodosum, aphthous, and episcleritis	Arthritis, erythema nodosum or pyoderma gangrenosum, iritis, and uveitis

to shortening, thickening, and narrowing of the colon. Complications include risk for toxic dilatation (toxic mega-colon) and dysplastic changes (carcinoma) of the intestine. Carcinoma of the colon is 10 times more likely in patients with ulcerative colitis than in the general population.

Physical Evaluation (See Table 4 –1)

Laboratory Studies
The diagnosis is made following colonoscopy, biopsy, and histologic examination of intestinal mucosal. Abdominal radiographs are also helpful.

Medical Treatment
Treatment of IBD involves the use of anti-inflammatory medications (sulfasalazine, 5-aminosalicylic acid, and cor-ticosteroids). If required, immunosuppressive agents and antibiotics are used next. Third-line approaches include monoclonal antibody (infliximab [Remicade]) against tumor necrosis factor or surgical resection.

Physical Status
IBD can range in severity (from American Society of Anes-thesiology (ASA) II to IV) based on the extent of the disease and level of control obtained by medical therapy. More severe disease leads to persistent pain, malabsorption, and anemia. Many patients will require surgical interventions at some time during the course of these lifelong diseases.

Dental Management
- Most patients with IBD have intermittent attacks, with asymptomatic remissions between attacks. Urgent dental care is advised only during acute exacerbations of gastrointestinal disease.
- Elective dental procedures should be scheduled during periods of remission when complications are absent.
- Patients who have IBD may be taking corticosteroids or immunosuppressant drugs that can affect oral health and dental management.
  - Most routine dental care can be performed without the need for additional corticosteroids. Adequate pain and anxiety control must be provided.
  - Supplemental corticosteroids are recommended for major stressful/surgical procedures when significant postoperative pain is anticipated. The guidelines for the provision of supplemental corti-costeroids are discussed in Chapter 3.
  - Blood studies (complete blood count with differential, liver function and renal function studies) should be obtained and reviewed for patients who take immunosuppressant drugs

(e.g., methotrexate) prior to invasive procedures. Abnormal results require delay in treatment and referral to a physician.
- For patients taking methotrexate, inquiries should be made as to the patient's breathing capacity as this drug can cause pulmonary fibrosis.
- A thorough head and neck examination should be performed on patients taking immunosuppres-sants because of the increased risk for lymphoma and infections [(e.g., infectious mononucleosis, recurrent herpes (see Figure 4 –1)].

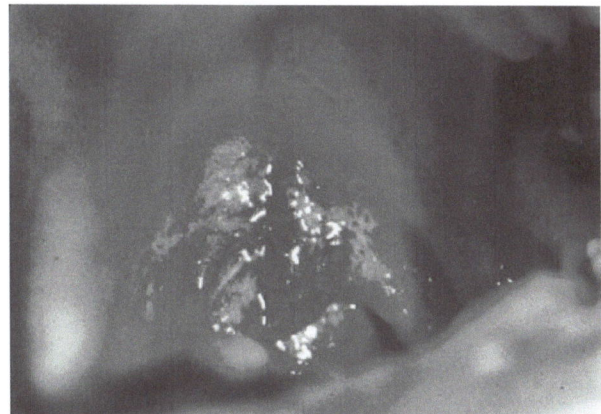

FIGURE 4-1: *Oral ulceration of the soft palate and uvula in a patient who had IBD.*

For pain relief, acetaminophen alone or in combination with opioids can be used. A careful drug history should be obtained to avoid prescribing additional opioids to patients taking these medications to manage their intestinal pain.

LIVER DISEASE
The patient with liver disease presents a significant management challenge for the dentist because the liver plays a vital role in metabolic functions, including the secretion of bile needed for fat absorption, conversion of sugar to glycogen, and excretion of bilirubin, a waste product of hemoglobin metabolism. Impairment of liver function can lead to abnormalities of the metabolism of amino acids, ammonia, protein, carbohydrates, and lipids (triglycerides and cholesterol). Many biochemical functions performed by the liver, such as synthesis of coagulation factors and drug metabolism (Table 4-2), may be adversely affected in the dental patient with acute or chronic liver disease. So along with impaired drug metabolism, significant bleeding may be a problem. Viral hepatitis and alcoholic liver disease are two of the more common liver disorders. In many cases, dysfunction of the liver will continue to progress over time. Therefore,

TABLE 4–2: Dental Drugs Metabolized Primarily by the Liver

Local anesthetics (appear safe for use during liver disease when used in appropriate amounts)	Analgesics	Sedatives
Lidocaine (Xylocaine) Mepivacaine (Carbocaine) Prilocaine (Citanest) Bupivacaine (Marcaine)	Aspirin* Acetaminophen (Tylenol, Datril) † Codeine† Meperidine (Demerol) † Ibuprofen (Motrin) *	Diazepam (Valium) † Barbiturates† **Antibiotics** Ampicillin Metronidazole ‡ Tetracycline Vancomycin ‡

* Limit dose or avoid if severe liver disease (acute hepatitis and cirrhosis) or hemostatic abnormalities are present.

† Limit dose or avoid if severe liver disease (acute hepatitis and cirrhosis) or encephalopathy is present or if taken with alcohol.

‡ Avoid if severe liver disease (acute hepatitis and cirrhosis) is present.

TABLE 4–3: Dental Management of the Patient with Alcoholic Liver Disease

1. Detection by such methods as
   History
   Clinical examination
   Alcohol odor on breath
   Information from family members or friends

2. Referral or consultation with physician to ascertain the following:
   Verify history
   Check current status
   Check medications
   Check laboratory values
   Discuss suggestions for management

3. Laboratory screening (if not available from physician) to record the following:
   Complete blood count with differential
   Alanine aminotransferase, Aspartate aminotransferase
   Bleeding time
   Thrombin time
   Prothrombin time

4. Assessment of risk of adverse outcome associated with invasive procedure or infection using prognostic formula (i.e., Modified Child-Pugh Classification found in table below)

Key Points			
Parameter	1	2	3
Ascites	None	Moderate	Severe
Encephalopathy	None	Mild (grade 1–2)	Severe (grade 3–4)
Serum bilirubin (mg/dL)	< 2.0	2.0–3.0	> 3.0
Serum albumin (mg/dL)	> 3.5	2.8–3.5	< 2.8
Prothrombin time (seconds increased)	1–3	4–6	> 6

Patients are scored by adding the numerical value obtained from each row and are then categorized as either class A (mild disease) = score 5 or 6; class B (moderate disease) = score of 7 to 9; or class C (severe disease)= score of 10 to 15.

5. Minimizing of drugs metabolized by liver (see Table 4-2)

6. If screening tests are abnormal, for surgical procedures, consider using thrombin, Gelfoam, antifibrinolytic agents, fresh frozen plasma, vitamin K, and platelets—with the help of a physician or PharmD.

TABLE 4–4: Features Associated with Advanced Alcoholic Liver
Systemic Complications
Traumatic or unexplained injuries (driving under the influence, bruises, cuts, scars, broken teeth)
Attention and memory deficits
Slurred speech
Spider angiomas
Jaundice (sclerae, mucosa)
Peripheral edema (edematous puffy face, ankle edema)
Ascites
Palmar erythema, white nails, or transverse pale band on nails
Ecchymoses, petechiae, or prolonged bleeding
Failure to fulfill role obligations at work, school, home (e.g., missed dental appointments)
Increased levels of bilirubin, aminotransferases, alkaline phosphates, γ-glutamyl transpeptidase, and mean corpuscular volume

for dental management. The kidneys regulate fluid volume and the acid-base balance of the plasma; excrete nitrogenous waste; synthesize erythropoietin, 1,25-dihydroxycholecalciferol, and renin; and are responsible for drug metabolism. The kidneys also are the target organ for parathormone and aldosterone. Progressive disease of the kidney can result in decreased function and manifestations in several organ systems. As a result, patient care can be impacted by the resulting anemia, abnormal bleeding, electrolyte and fluid imbalance, hypertension, drug intolerance, and skeletal abnormalities. In addition, patients who have severe and progressive disease may require artificial filtration of the blood by dialysis or transplantation of a kidney.

Definition

Renal disease is a progressive destruction of the kidney tissues that can lead to a complete shutdown in the kidney's ability to excrete urine and secrete important hormones. The terminology associated with kidney diseases includes nephritic syndrome, end-stage renal disease, azotemia, uremic syndrome, and advanced renal disease.

Etiology

Acute renal failure is most often the result of acute renal disease or an ischemic insult to the kidney, caused by trauma, toxic agents, certain drugs, septicemia, or premature separation of the placenta. Chronic renal failure most often results from underlying abnormalities of the kidney or is secondary to systemic disease. Causes of chronic renal failure include chronic glomerulonephritis, hypertension, diabetes mellitus, chronic pyelonephritis, polycystic disease, and drug-induced nephropathies. Long-term abuse

patients with liver disorders are of significant importance to the dentist, and require proper management.

RENAL DISEASE

Chronic renal disease and its ultimate result, end-stage renal disease (ESRD), are a worldwide problem and continue to increase. Since patients with ESRD have many serious medical problems, dentists must know how to properly manage them. This chapter reviews the current status of ESRD and presents the principles

TABLE 4–5: Clinical Findings Associated with Renal Disease	
Organ System	**Common Systemic Manifestations**
Neuromuscular	Lethargy, mental slowness, lassitude, weakness
Cardiovascular	Hypertension, pericarditis, cardiomyopathy, congestive heart failure
Alpha-glucosidase inhibitors	Decrease carbohydrate absorption, preventing a rise in glucose after meals
Dermatologic	Pruritus, exaggerated bruising, hyperpigmentation
Hematologic	Increased bleeding time, lymphopenia, increased susceptibility to infection, anemia (owing to decreased secretion of erythropoietin)
Metabolic	Glucose intolerance, lipid abnormalities
Endocrinologic	The parathyroid glands are stimulated and cause a number of changes. These can be manifested radiologically in several ways, including generalized radiolucencies of the bones or jaw radiolucencies.
*It is estimated that 90% of the kidney can be nonfunctional, yet it can still perform its daily activities in a nonstressed environment.	

TABLE 4–6: Common Tests to Aid with the Diagnosis of Renal Disease	
Diagnostic Test	**How Test Is Evaluated**
Glomerular filtration rate	Normal range = 120 cc/min (SI Units= 2); can drop to 10 cc/min (SI = 0.15) or lower in chronic renal failure
Blood area nitrogen	The normal level is less than 20 mg/100 mL (SI Units = 7); level increased bleeding can rise if this level reaches above 50 mg/100 mL (SI = 18)
Creatinine level	The normal level is less than 1.5 mg/100 mL (SI Units = 135). Systemic problems can arise if this level exceeds 5 mg/100 mL (SI = 440).
Electrolytes	Hyperkalemic and hypocalcemic conditions may be present, which could lead to cardiac arrhythmia
Urinalysis	To be analyzed are specific gravity, osmolality, pH, and presence of abnormal constituents (protein, blood, etc.)
Radiographic examination	Can demonstrate calcification and size and contour of kidneys
Ultrasonographic examination	Can demonstrate tumors, cysts, obstruction, and polycystic kidney disease.
Renal biopsy	Can demonstrate pathologic changes associated with acute or chronic disease
SI = International Standard Units.	

of over-the-counter analgesics, especially acetaminophen, can exacerbate chronic renal failure.

Clinical Findings/Presentation
Chronic renal failure is a gradual ongoing loss of nephron function for which nephron hypertrophy is unable to compensate. It is generally asymptomatic at first; however, there is later significant impairment of all renal function with effects on virtually all body systems.

Evaluation/Diagnosis
Disease of the kidney is identified by clinical symptoms and by evaluation of the functioning status of the kidney through imaging and evaluation of blood chemistries and urine analysis (Table 4 – 6).
- Renal insufficiency: Early phase characterized by nocturia and anorexia
- Renal failure: Late phase characterized by a myriad of signs and symptoms, depending on the organ system

Medical Management
Treatment of severe and acute renal failure, if the duration is prolonged for more than several days, generally aims at stabilization by rigid control of fluid electrolytes and acid-base balance. Dialysis will be used. Treatment of chronic renal failure in the early stages is conservative, with a strict diet and electrolyte control. In later stages, dialysis is required, with some individual candidates for renal transplantation. Advanced renal disease is usually treated by dialysis (either hemodialysis or peritoneal dialysis) and/or kidney transplantation.

Hemodialysis
Metabolic wastes are removed by passing the patient's blood through thin, semipermeable membranes to filter the waste products. The blood is heparinized and then returned to the patient. An arteriovenous fistula is usually made for long-term dialysis patients.

Peritoneal Dialysis
Used in advanced renal disease, peritoneal dialysis is slower and the abdominal peritoneum acts as the filter. The waste fluid is drained from the abdomen after a specific period.

Renal Transplantation
The organ transplant can be from a relative, unrelated but matched donor, or cadaver donor. Because of tissue matching and the waiting time for a cadaver kidney, a kidney transplant from a relative is preferable. All transplant patients are placed on a lifetime regimen of immunosuppressive drugs.

Dental Management of the Patient with ESRD (Including Emergency Dental Care)

Conservative Care
- Consult with physician regarding physical status and level of control.

- Avoid dental treatment if disease is unstable (poorly controlled or advanced).
- Screen for bleeding disorder before surgery (bleeding time, platelet count, hematocrit, hemoglobin).
- Monitor blood pressure closely.
- Pay meticulous attention to good surgical technique.
- Avoid nephrotoxic drugs (acetaminophen in high doses, acyclovir, aspirin, nonsteroidal anti-inflammatory drugs, tetracycline).
- Adjust dosage of drugs metabolized by the kidney (see Table 4-8).
- Manage orofacial infections aggressively with culture and sensitivity test and antibiotics.
- Consider hospitalization for severe infection or major procedures.
- Consider corticosteroid supplementation as indicated.

Receiving Hemodialysis
- Same as conservative care recommendations.
- Beware of concerns of arteriovenous shunt.
- Avoid blood pressure cuff and IV medications in arm with shunt.
- Avoid dental care on day of hemodialysis treatment (especially within first 6 hours afterward); best to treat on day after.
- Consider antimicrobial prophylaxis (based on guidelines).
- Consider corticosteroid supplementation as indicated.

Assess status of liver function and presence of opportunistic infection in these patients because of increased risk for carrier state of hepatitis B and C viruses and human immunodeficiency virus (HIV).

ORAL HEALTH CARE CONSIDERATIONS
A thorough history of renal disease, including etiology and extent of organ systems affected, knowledge of laboratory tests specific to kidney functions, and an understanding of the various treatment modalities, aids in optimal oral health care. The dentist must be aware that the normal warning signs of inflammation and infection may be masked. The patient with ESRD can present with a multitude of problems to the oral health care provider. Good communication and consultation with the patient's physician concerning therapy, prophylactic antibiotic coverage, and specific laboratory tests are recommended before initiating invasive dental procedures.

CLINICIAN TIPS:
- Most hemodialysis patients undergo dialysis three times a week.
- The best time to provide dental care is the day after the dialysis session.
- Be aware of possible immunosuppression and adrenal insufficiency in post–renal transplantation patients.

TABLE 4–7: Pharmacologic Management	
Considerations	*Management*
Compromised excretion of drug	Careful adjustment of dosages and intervals of dosage. Review drug interaction and site of drug clearance.
Patients undergoing dialysis	Careful attention to avoid drugs not dialyzed (consult hospital pharmacy)
Drug nephrotoxicity	Careful attention to published drug guidelines (consult hospital pharmacy)
Antibiotic therapy	Avoid nephrotoxic drugs, especially aminoglycosides (streptomycin, gentamicin, neomycin) and polypeptides (polymyxin B). Tetracyclines can cause dangerous increase in blood urea nitrogen.
Analgesic therapy	Salicylates can be nephrotoxic. Salicylates and NSAIDs may cause bleeding or excess fluid retention. Long-term NSAID therapy is to be avoided.
NSAID = nonsteroidal anti-inflammatory drug.	

TABLE 4 – 8: Adjustment of Drugs During Renal Failure					
Drug	Elimination and Metabolism	Removal by Dialysis	> 50	GFR, mL/min 10 – 50	< 10
Analgesic					
Aspirin	Liver (kidney)	Yes	q4h	q6h	Avoid
Acetaminophen	Liver	Yes	q4h	q6h	q8h
Ibuprofen (Motrin)		?	Normal dosing	Normal dosing	Normal dosing
Propoxyphene* (Darvon)	Liver (kidney)	No	Normal dosing	75% dose	Avoid
Codeine	Liver	?	Normal dosing	75% dose	50% dose
Meperidine* (Dermerol	Liver	?	Normal dosing	75% dose	50% dose
Anesthetic					
Lidocaine (Xylocaine)	Liver (kidney)	No	q12h	Normal dosing	Normal dosing
Antimicrobial					
Acyclovir (Zovirax)	Kidney	Yes	q8h	q12-24h	50% dose q12-24h
Amoxicillin, penicillin V	Kidney (liver)	No	q8h	q8-12h	q24h
Cephalexin (Keflex)	Kidney	Yes	q8h	q12h	q12h
Clindamycin (Cleocin)	Liver	No	Normal dosing	Normal dosing	Normal dosing
Erythromycin	Liver	No	Normal dosing	Normal dosing	50-70% dose
Ketoconazole (Nizoral)	Liver	No	Normal dosing	Normal dosing	Normal dosing
Metronidazole (Flagyl)	Liver (Kidney)	Yes	Normal dosing	Normal dosing	50% dose
Tetracycline (Doxycycline)	Kidney (Liver)	No	q8h-12h	q12-24h	q24h
Benzodiazepine					
Diazepam (Valium) Triazolam (Halcion)	Liver	?	Normal dosing	Normal dosing	Normal dosing
Corticosteroid					
Dexamethasone	Locally & Liver		Normal dosing	Normal dosing	Normal dosing

Adapted from Proctor R et al. Oral and dental aspects of chronic renal failure. J Dent Res 2005;84:199–208; and Singh G. Renal disease. Med Clin North Am 2005;89:240.

DR = dosage reduction; GFR = glomerular filtration rate; HD = hemodialysis; I = increase interval between doses; NA = not available; PD = peritoneal dialysis.

*Have toxic metabolites that can build up in severe ESRD.

TABLE 4 –9: Primary Laboratory Values for the Assessment of Renal Function and Failure			
Laboratory Test	Reference Value	Indicator of Renal Insufficiency	Indicator of Renal Failure
Urine			
Creatinine clearance	85 – 125 mL/min (women) 97 – 140 mL/min (men)	50 – 90 mL/min 50 – 90 mL/min	10 – 50 mL/min (moderate) <10 mL/min (severe)
Glomerular filtration rate (GFR)	100 - 150 mL/min		10 – 50 mL/min (moderate) <10 mL/min (severe)
Serum			
Blood urea nitrogen (BUN)	8 – 18 mg/dL	20 – 30 mg/dL	30 – 50 mg/dL (moderate) >50 mg/dL (severe)
Creatinine	0.6 – 1.20 mg/dL	2 – 3 mg/dL	3 – 6 mg/dL (moderate) >6 mg/dL (severe)

Adapted from Zachee P, Vermylen J, Boogaerts MA. Ann Hematol 1994;69:33–40; and De Rossi SS, Glick M. Dental considerations for the patient with renal disease receiving hemodialysis. J Am Dent Assoc 1996;127:211–9.

Secondary indicators of renal function. Normal reference values: calcium 8.2 to 11.2 mg/dL; chloride 95 to 103 mmol/L; inorganic phosphorus 2.7 to 4.5 mg/dL; potassium 3.8 to 5 mmol/L; sodium 136 to 142 mmol/L; total carbon dioxide for venous blood 22 to 26 mmol/L.

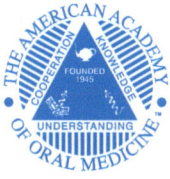

5 Hematology

BLEEDING DISORDERS

Sources of bleeding disorders are multiple and a comprehensive discussion of them and their management is beyond the scope of this monograph. Included in this discussion are the most commonly detected findings that are relevant to dentistry.

Identification of Patients with Potential Bleeding Problems

Listed in Table 5-1 are some of the more commonly observed findings from the subjective/objective examination that should alert the clinician to a potential bleeding problem.

Tests of Hemostasis

Tables 5-2 and 5-3 are summary tables of basic diagnostic testing for a number of coagulation and platelet disorders. The sophistication and multiplicity of available tests often require joint patient management with the patient's hematologist.

TABLE 5–1: Examination Findings Suggestive of Potential Bleeding Problems	
Objective/Physical	*Subjective/Health History*
Prolonged bleeding after trauma/surgery	History of bleeding problems
Spontaneous bleeding	Medications (coumarin warfarin, heparin, aspirin, other anticoagulant and
Epistaxis	antiplatelet agents)
Petechiae/ecchymosis	Liver disease/hepatitis
Jaundice/ascites	Cirrhosis
Spider angiomas	Renal failure
Severe anemia	Hemophilia A, B, C
Hemarthrosis	von Willebrand disease
Telangiectasias	Alcohol abuse
Abnormal laboratory tests	Current cancer treatment

Coagulation Phase Measures

TABLE 5–2: Laboratory Tests of Coagulation Phase		
Test	*Normal**	*Purpose*
Prothrombin time (PT)	11–14 s	Measures extrinsic coagulation pathway Prolonged with deficiencies of factors II, V, VII, and X and fibrinogen
International normalized ratio (INR)	< 1.1	Adjusts PT values for sensitivity of laboratory's reagents using formula INR = {patient's PT/control PT}^{ISI}, where ISI[†] is reagent adjustment
Activated partial thromboplastin time	30–40 s	Measures intrinsic pathway; detects deficiencies of factors II, V, VIII, IX, X, XI, XII
Thrombin time	9–13 s	Detects circulating inhibitors, decreased fibrinogen, or dysfibrinogenemia
*Control values are approximate only. Patient values should be compared with the controls for the laboratory used. [†] ISI values for commercial thromboplastins used in the United States range from 1.2 to 2.8.		

TABLE 5–3: Laboratory Tests of Platelet Phase		
Functional Measures of Platelet Activity	*Normal**	*Purpose*
Ivy bleeding time	< 7 min	An in vivo test of platelet function that detects quantitative and qualitative platelet defects such as von Willebrand disease and thrombocytopenia
Platelet function analyzer 100 (PFA-100, Dade Behring Inc., Deerfield, IL)	Closure time <180s	Quantitative laboratory measurement of platelet function; avoids variability of bleeding time

Platelet Phase Measures

The normal platelet count range is 150,000 to 400,000 cells/mL. A clinical bleeding problem may occur below 80,000 cells/mL, and replacement therapy for surgical procedures may be necessary at less than 50,000 cells/mL. The platelet count gives the number of thrombocytes, but it does not tell whether they are functioning properly.

POTENTIAL BLEEDING DISORDERS
ACQUIRED COAGULOPATHIES

Patients Taking Coumarin

Coumarin anticoagulation such as warfarin (Coumadin), prescribed to approximately 1 million individuals in the United States each year, is the most likely bleeding problem that dentists encounter. Coumarin is prescribed to prevent venous thrombosis and systemic embolism in susceptible patients. The duration of therapy varies from short periods to the remainder of the patient's life. For most indications, the international normalized ratio (INR) range goal is from 2.0 to 3.0. Individuals with mechanical heart valves are usually kept in an INR range of 2.5 to 3.5. There are a few, relatively rare, indications for anticoagulation with coumarin with an INR above 3.5.

Coumarin acts as a vitamin K antimetabolite, thereby interfering with the synthesis of factors VII, IX, and X and prothrombin. After oral administration, coumarin usually takes 4 to 5 days for adequate anticoagulation to be achieved. Because of absorption irregularities, the degree of anticoagulation can vary despite the dosage remaining constant. Most patients are monitored at least monthly to make sure the desired level of anticoagulation is achieved and maintained.

Dental Patient Assessment

During the initial evaluation of a patient taking coumarin, dentists should pursue two courses of evaluation: a detailed interview of the patient and a patient needs assessment (Table 5-4).

Laboratory Testing

The primary effect of coumarin is in the common pathway owing to the inadequate amounts of prothrombin. When evaluating a patient taking coumarin, the appropriate test is the prothrombin time (PT) or INR. Ideally, testing should be done within 24 hours of scheduled dental treatment. To save cost and inconvenience to the patient, it is desirable for the dentist to schedule his or her treatment at a time when the physician would normally monitor the patient. Practitioners who see many patients taking coumarin may want to consider purchase of the in-office CoaguChek (Roche Diagnostics, Indianapolis, IN) system for monitoring INR.

Dental Management

Dental care for a patient receiving coumarin therapy requires balancing the opposing risks of significant hemorrhage from dental procedures against the potential for thromboembolism from reduced or withdrawn therapy (Figures 5- 1 and 5-2). In consultation, the physician and dentist should jointly decide the best management strategy based on a hemorrhagic risk assessment. Complete cessation of anticoagulation therapy for dental treatment is not indicated.

TABLE 5–4: Dental Evaluation of the Patient Taking Coumarin	
Patient Interview	*Patient Needs Assessment*
Name of the attending physician	Types of dental therapy required
Reason for coumarin therapy	Potential for hemorrhage
Anticipated duration of therapy	Presence of local factors that increase the potential for hemorrhage
Frequency of monitoring	Necessity for block anesthesia
Stability of therapy	Number of anticipated visits

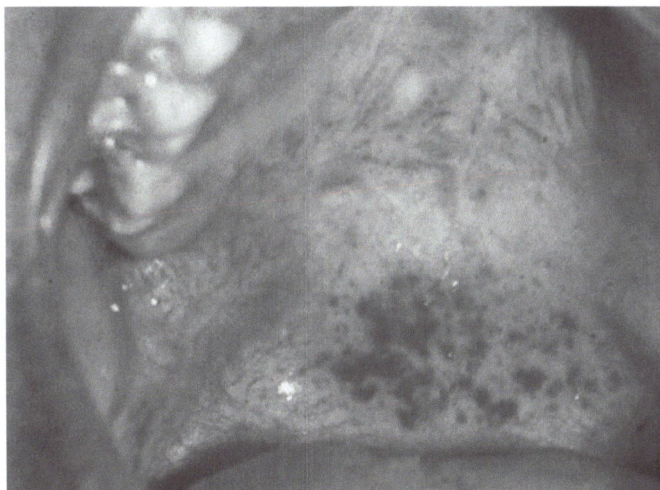

FIGURE 5 -1: *Ecchymosis on the palate of a patient with a bleeding disorder as a result of Coumadin therapy.*

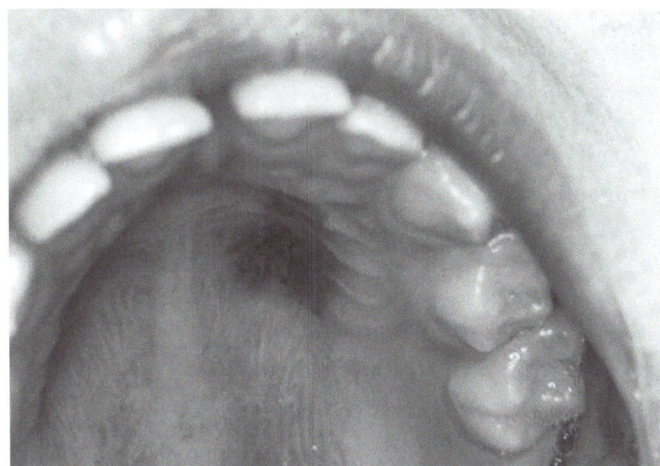

FIGURE 5 -2: *Ecchymosis on the palate of a patient with a bleeding disorder as a result of Coumadin therapy.*

If the duration of anticoagulation therapy is anticipated to be 6 months or less, providers may want to postpone elective care until after normal cessation of therapy. This is especially true if non-urgent surgery is part of the proposed treatment.

It is essential to evaluate the patient as described above and to have a current INR available prior to treatment. There is good empiric evidence that all but the most extensive **dental care can be safely performed as long as the patient's INR is below 3.5.** Hemorrhage can be controlled with local measures such as mechanical procedures (sutures, pressure), chemical agents (thrombin, tranexamic acid), and absorbable hemostatic agents (oxidized cellulose, microfibrillar hemostat).

For extensive treatment such as full-mouth extraction, treatment management options include dividing the planned surgeries into smaller segments done separately or possibly shifting the patient to the lower range of anticoagulation by withholding coumarin for 2 to 3 days. Another option would be to switch the patient from coumarin to heparin and then discontinue the heparin for a short period of time (6–8 hours), perform the surgery, and resume anticoagulation with coumarin. This intensive shifting of anticoagulation regimens often requires hospitalization, but with the newer low-molecular-weight heparins (LMWHs), which can be self-administered subcutaneously, the procedure can be accomplished on an outpatient basis. All alterations of anticoagulation therapy must be done by the patient's physician in consultation with the treating dentist.

Caution

The anticoagulation effect of coumarin can be substantially increased by antibiotic therapy. If antibiotics are employed as part of treatment, periodic monitoring of INR is recommended. Patients on coumarin therapy should not be prescribed aspirin or nonsteroidal anti-inflammatory drugs (NSAIDs) because of their increased bleeding potential.

Patients Taking Heparin

Heparin acts as an antithromboplastin, preventing the enzymatic conversion of prothrombin to thrombin. It is used predominantly in a hospital environment. Heparin is given intravenously and has a brief duration of action (4 hours). Patient status can be monitored using the activated partial thromboplastin time (aPTT). However, in the majority of instances, dental treatment is deferred until the patient is no longer on this medication.

Heparin is commonly used in renal dialysis treatment. Normally, one would not treat patients requiring hemodialysis on the same day as their therapy because of the increased potential for bleeding with the use of heparin.

With the increased use of the newer LMWHs (enoxaparin [Lovenox, Sanofi-Aventis, Bridgewater, NJ], dalteparin [Fragmin]), it is much more likely that patients receiving heparin will be seen on an outpatient basis. Indications for LMWHs include outpatient treatment of deep vein thrombosis and prophylaxis in high risk patients such as those undergoing hip or knee replacement surgery or abdominal surgery. Advantages of LMWH include once-a-day dosing, potential home treatment, and a more predictable effect on anticoagulation. Consultation with the prescribing physician is necessary before recommending cessation for dental care.

Patients Taking Other Anticoagulants

Dabigatran (Pradaxa) is a direct thrombin inhibitor while rivaroxaban (Xarelto), apixaban (Eliquis) and edoxaban (Savaysa) are direct factor Xa inhibitors. These newer anticoagulants are indicated for the prevention of stroke in nonvalvular atrial fibrillation and for the prophylaxis of deep vein thrombosis or pulmonary embolism following orthopedic surgery. Unlike coumarin anticoagulants, these drugs are not routinely monitored by coagulation assays.

For most dental procedures with mild to moderate risk of bleeding, discontinuation of these anticoagulant agents is typically unwarranted. For extensive surgery with high risk of bleeding, consultation with the patient's physician is necessary to evaluate the need to reduce or withhold anticoagulation. Therapy may be withheld for 1-2 days prior to the procedure based on the creatinine clearance. For all procedures, atraumatic surgical techniques and local measures should be used to control hemorrhage.

Other Acquired Causes Of Coagulation Deficiencies

Additional acquired causes of coagulation deficiencies include severe liver disease, cirrhosis, malabsorption syndrome, celiac disease, long-term antibiotic therapy, and biliary tract obstruction.

CONGENITAL COAGULATION FACTOR DEFICIENCIES

Hemophilias

The sex-linked recessive disorders of hemophilia A and B occur in approximately 1 in 5,000 and 1 in 30,000 male births, respectively. It is estimated that there are more 20,000 individuals with hemophilia in the United States. Because of its hereditary aspect, concentration in certain geographic areas occurs. Hemophilia A is a factor VIII deficiency (antihemophilic globulin) and accounts for 80% of all genetic coagulation disorders. Hemophilia B (Christmas disease) is a factor IX deficiency (plasma thromboplastin component) and accounts for 13% of genetic coagulation disorders.

Although almost all hemophiliac patients are male, it is possible for females to be affected. Patients with hemophilia A or B often present with similar clinical presentations. Clinical severity is inversely proportional to the circulating levels of factors VIII and IX. Severe deficiency is less than 1% of normal. Spontaneous bleeds are uncommon with 5% or greater of normal activity. Approximately 60% of all cases of hemophilia A are severe, whereas only 20 to 45%

of hemophilia B is severe.

Medical Management

Prevention and reversal of acute bleeding events involve replacement of the missing or deficient clotting factor. Replacement guidelines strive to obtain plasma levels at 25 to 30% activity for minor spontaneous or traumatic bleeds. For treatment or prevention of severe bleeds, including major dental surgery, a level of > 50% activity is necessary. A large number of clotting factor concentrates for hemophilia A and B are available in the United States. Also available and very useful are antifibrinolytic agents. Agents such as Amicar, ε-aminocaproic acid (EACA), desmopressin, and tranexamic acid help maintain the fibrin meshwork that is formed during hemostasis. In many instances, the administration of these agents is sufficient by itself and factor replacement is not required.

GENERAL GUIDELINES FOR DENTAL TREATMENT
- Work closely with the hematologist
- Be familiar with the type and severity of disease
- Limit bleeding
- Use block anesthesia with caution
- Avoid aspirin
- Protect soft tissue
- Never compromise the quality of dental care

GUIDELINES FOR DENTAL SURGERY
- The emphasis is on prevention of the anticipated bleeding
- Describe specific treatment to the hematologist
- Obtain adequate factor replacement as needed
- Use antifibrinolytic agents as necessary
- Use local hemostatic measures
- Follow post-extraction for bleeding

GUIDELINES FOR REMOVAL OF DECIDUOUS TEETH
- Allow for natural exfoliation
- Use topical hemostatic agents as necessary
- Treat with antifibrinolytic agents/factor replacement as necessary

Von Willebrand Disease (Pseudohemophilia)

von Willebrand disease (vWD), which results from a deficiency of von Willebrand factor (vWF), is the most common inherited bleeding disorder, with a prevalence of 1% of the general population. Both sexes are affected equally, and there is no ethnic predilection. Three major types of the disease are recognized based on phenotypic classification, types 1, 2 and 3. Type 2 has various subtypes. Many individuals with vWD have mild disease and remain undiagnosed

TABLE 5–5: Conditions Associated with Decreased Thrombocytopoiesis	
General Causes of Decreased Production	**Specific Conditions Associated with Decreased Thrombocytopoiesis**
Hypoplasia of hematopoietic stem cells	Aplastic anemia Marrow damage from ionizing radiation, alcohol, drugs, chemicals, infections Congenital and hereditary thrombocytopenias
Marrow replacement	Leukemias Metastatic cancers from breast/prostate, lymphoma
Ineffective thrombocytopoiesis	Vitamin B12 (cobalamin) or folate deficiency Hematopoietic dysplastic syndromes

until trauma or surgery. Associated symptoms include easy bruising, mucosal surface bleeding, epistaxis, gastrointestinal hemorrhage, and menorrhagia. vWD is associated clinically with Osler-Weber-Rendu syndrome.

Laboratory Testing
The bleeding time, PFA-100 test, and aPTT are variably prolonged. The vWF activity assay or ristocetin cofactor activity (vWF:RCoF) is the most specific test for vWF function but may be only slightly increased in mild vWD.

Medical Management
The therapeutic goal is to correct deficiencies in vWF activity to > 50% of normal with factor VIII activity at appropriate levels for the clinical situation. Desmopressin and adjunctive use of antifibrinolytic agents such as epsilon aminocaproic acid or tranexamic acid are also employed as necessary.

GUIDELINES FOR DENTAL TREATMENT
See Hemophilia above.

OTHER CONGENITAL COAGULATION DEFICIENCIES
Another potential congenital coagulation deficiency is hemophilia C (factor XI deficiency plasma thromboplastin antecedent). Effectively any of the components of the coagulation cascade can have deficiency status. Consultation with the attending physician is essential. Generally, the dentist should follow protocols similar to those described above for hemophiliacs.

Thrombocytopenias
Platelets provide both mechanical blockage of bleeding sites and releasing platelet factors that activate or complement the coagulation cascade. Low platelet levels (thrombocytopenias) can be produced by a diverse assortment of etiologies. In general, these etiologies can be classified as disturbances in production, increased destruction, or distribution problems. Distribution problems refer to hypersplenism and platelet pooling within the spleen secondary to congestive splenomegaly, Gaucher disease, and lymphoma. Thrombocytopenia owing to decreased production can develop from hypoplasia of hematopoietic stem cells from either an overall decrease in cellularity or infiltration by abnormal cells. Decreased production of platelets also results from abnormal maturation of megakaryocytes and resultant decreased thrombocytopoiesis. Table 5-5 lists some of the disorders associated with decreased production of thrombocytes.

TABLE 5–6: Conditions Associated with Increased Platelet Destruction	
General Causes of Increased Platelet Destruction	**Specific Conditions Associated with Increased Platelet Destruction**

Immune disorders	Idiopathic thrombocytopenia purpura
	Secondary to
	  Cancer (chronic lymphocytic leukemia, lymphoma)
	  Systemic autoimmune disease (SLE, polyarteritis nodosa) Infectious
	  diseases (infectious mononucleosis, CMV, HIV)
	  Over 50 drugs, including quinine, quinidine, heparin, sulfa compounds,
	  thiazide diuretics, penicillin

Nonimmune disorders	Disseminated intravascular coagulation
CMV = cytomegalovirus; HIV = human immunodeficiency virus; SLE = systemic lupus erythematosus.	

Increased destruction of platelets results from a variety of both immunologic and nonimmune disorders. A classic example of an autoimmune-mediated bleeding disorder is idiopathic thrombocytopenia purpura (ITP), characterized by development of antibodies to one's own platelets. The diagnosis of ITP is dependent on exclusion of other underlying systemic disorders that can result in thrombocytopenia. Table 5-6 lists some of the disorders associated with increased destruction of platelets.

Medical Management
Treatment of thrombocytopenia is initially directed toward identifying the cause through an algorithm of history, physical examination, and laboratory testing. If an underlying cause is identified, management of the underlying cause can sometimes reverse the thrombocytopenia. In other instances, care focuses on bleeding prevention and adjunctive care with surgery. Prednisone therapy, splenectomy, and intravenous gammaglobulin are used as necessary. Platelet transfusions are effective for some indications, but repeated transfusions stimulate alloantibodies.

Laboratory Testing
Testing usually consists of monitoring platelet counts. Patients with platelet counts of 100,000/µL or higher rarely have abnormal bleeding even with major surgery. With a platelet count of 20,000 to 50,000/µL, bleeding occurs with minor trauma and spontaneous bleeding occurs below 20,000/µL.

Functional Inadequacies of Platelets
Functional defects of platelets can arise from both congenital and acquired causes.

ACQUIRED FUNCTIONAL PLATELET DEFECTS
Aspirin is used in medicine for many purposes, including prevention of thrombosis. Ingestion of aspirin results in the irreversible inhibition of the enzyme cyclooxygenase, which is required for the synthesis of thromboxane A2 and prostaglandins. This effect persists for the life of the thrombocyte (approximately 9 days). NSAIDs also inhibit cyclooxygenase, but this effect is reversible on withdrawal.

Ticlopidine hydrochloride (Ticlid) and clopidogrel (Plavix) are used to reduce atherosclerotic events (myocardial infarction, stroke, vascular deaths). They inhibit platelet aggregation by interfering with adenosine diphosphate (ADP)-induced platelet-fibrinogen binding and subsequent platelet-platelet interactions. Their effect on platelet function is irreversible for the life of the platelet.

Fibrinogen receptor (platelet cell surface glycoproteins IIb and IIIa) inhibitors are available as tirofiban (Aggrastat), abciximab (ReoPro), and eptifibatide (Integrilin).

Dipyridamole (Persantine) increases cyclic adenosine monophosphate and was once used as a single therapy for anticoagulation therapy. This use was found to be ineffective; however, it is still being used as adjunct with warfarin to decrease thrombosis in patients after artificial heart valves; and combining with aspirin for secondary prophylaxis of transient ischemic attack or cerebrovascular accident (marketed as Aggrenox).

Dental Management
Patients taking aspirin, NSAIDs, ADP and fibrinogen receptor inhibitors, and dipyridamole can have invasive dental procedures performed without altering the dosage. Any excessive bleeding can be controlled by local measures. If there is concern, a bleeding time can be taken. If the bleeding time is less than 20 minutes, it is safe to proceed. Aspirin should not be prescribed to patients taking ticlopidine hydrochloride or clopidogrel.

Caution
When agents reducing the functionality of platelets are combined with anticoagulants, the hemostatic mechanism is compromised on two fronts, and the dentist should take this into account when planning therapy.

OTHER CAUSES OF FUNCTIONAL INADEQUACIES IN PLATELETS
Uremia also produces functional abnormalities in platelets. The cause for this is not well understood. Dentists should work closely with the patient's nephrologist when managing with patients with end-stage renal disease. Alcohol can sometimes impair platelet function. The effect is proportional to the degree of alcohol ingestion. Numerous medications can also influence the functional capacities of platelets, but these effects are rarely sufficient to be clinically significant to the dental practitioner.

CONGENITAL CAUSES OF FUNCTIONAL INADEQUACIES IN PLATELETS
The congenital causes of functional inadequacies in platelets are grouped into three categories.

1. Defects of adhesion (Bernard-Soulier syndrome)

2. Defective platelet aggregation (Glanzmann thrombasthenia)

3. Disorders of platelet secretion (storage pool disorders)

TABLE 5–7: Basic Functions of White Blood Cell Subsets	
Subset	**Function**
Lymphoid lineage	Acquired immune response
T lymphocyte	Destruction of infected cells and antigen presentation to B cells
B lymphocyte	Antibody production
Natural killer cell	Destruction of virally infected cells and tumor cells
Myeloid lineage	Innate immune response
Neutrophil	Phagocytosis of foreign cells and bacteria
Eosinophil	Allergic responses and defense against helminth pathogens
Basophil	Mediators of immediate allergic and inflammatory responses
Monocyte	Phagocytosis and specialized antigen-presenting cells

Fortunately, all of these conditions are rare. When managing these patients, it is advised to work with the patient's hematologist. Platelet transfusion is often necessary.

WHITE BLOOD CELL DISORDERS

The WBC can be either increased or decreased, both of which can have important consequences to oral health and providing dental care. Leukocytosis is an abnormal increase in the WBC resulting from reactive or neoplastic disorders. Leukopenias are defined as a decrease in the WBC.

Hematopoietic Stem Cell Differentiation of White Blood Cells

White blood cells are a group of cells that differentiate from hematopoietic stem cells in the bone marrow and are primarily involved in the immune response. Division of these stem cells leads to the white blood cell lymphoid and myeloid lineages. Mature lymphoid cells include T lymphocytes, B lymphocytes, and natural killer cells, whereas mature myeloid cells include neutrophils, eosinophils, basophils, and monocytes. The functions of these white blood cells are described in Table 5-7.

Laboratory Tests to Evaluate White Blood Cell Disorders

The total WBC is one component of a CBC. The differential WBC represents the percent breakdown of the different subsets of white blood cells: lymphocytes, neutrophils, monocytes, eosinophils, and basophils. The absolute count for the different subsets of white blood cells can provide vital information for the clinical management of immunocompromised patients. For example, if a

TABLE 5–8: Basic Laboratory Tests Used to Evaluate WBCS	
Test	**Normal**
White blood cells (1,000/µL)	5.0–11
Differential WBC (%)	
Lymphocytes	10–45
Neutrophils	45–75
Monocytes	5–10
Eosinophils	0–5
Basophils	0–1
Bands (immature neutrophils)	0–5

patient has a WBC of 10,000/µL and the differential report indicates that 25% of the white blood cells are lymphocytes, then the absolute lymphocyte count (ALC) is 10,000/µL x 0.25 = 2,500/µL. In another example, the absolute neutrophil count (ANC) can be determined by adding the neutrophils and the bands (immature neutrophils). Therefore, if a patient had 10,000/µL white blood cells with 45% neutrophils and 5% bands, then 50% of all white blood cells are neutrophils, providing an ANC of 10,000/µL x 0.5 = 5,000/µL (see Table 5-8).

An elevated or decreased WBC is often related to the proliferation or deficiency of a particular subset of white blood cells. A deficiency in lymphocytes is termed lymphopenia, and a decrease in neutrophils is termed neutropenia. A quantitative increase of lymphocytes is termed lymphocytosis and an increase of neutrophils is termed neutrophilia.

TABLE 5–9: Selected Examples of Etiology of Leukopenia	
Etiology	*Examples*
Neutropenia (↓ neutrophils)	
Medications	Cytotoxic drugs; Antibiotics; Anti-inflammatory
Vitamin deficiency	Vitamin B12; Folic acid
Hematopoietic disorder	Leukemia; Aplastic anemia; Myelodysplasia; Other malignancies with bone marrow involvement
Underlying medical conditions	Viral infection; Autoimmune disease; Cyclic neutropenia; Hypersplenism; Advanced HIV infection (AIDS)
Lymphopenia (↓ lymphocytes)	
Infectious disease	HIV infections (AIDS); Acute viral infection
Drugs	Glucocorticoids; Cytotoxic drugs
Underlying medical condition	Autoimmune disease; Malnutrition; Di George syndrome; Bruton disease (X-linked agammaglobulinemia); Selective IgA deficiency; Severe combined immunodeficiency

LEUKOPENIA

A deficient WBC can be associated with numerous etiologies. A decrease in neutrophils is most commonly the etiology for a low WBC. Lymphopenia is less commonly the underlying etiology of a low WBC. A neutropenia is present with an ANC < 1,500/μL, with a severe neutropenia being <500/μL.

General Findings Associated with Leukopenia

The physical findings and symptoms of leukopenia are primarily associated with an increased risk of microbial infection. The risk of bacterial and fungal infection significantly increases when the ANC falls below 500/μL. (see Table 5-9).

Oral Manifestations

The oral manifestations can alert clinicians to suspect a low WBC and to obtain a CBC with differential to rule out this possibility. Oral findings that may be indicative of leukopenia include a Candida infection (pseudomembranous candidiasis, erythematous candidiasis, hyperplastic candidiasis, or angular cheilitis), deep fungal infection (e.g. histoplasmosis, mucormycosis, or aspergillosis), rapidly advancing periodontal disease, oral ulcerations, and recurrent oral viral infections. Although recurrent herpes simplex oral infection primarily affects the attached mucosa, these lesions can manifest on unattached mucosa with the presence of severe immunosuppression (see Table 5-10).

TABLE 5–10: Findings Associated with Leukopenia	
Objective/Physical Findings	*Subjective/Health History*
Lymphadenopathy Fever Skin rashes, redness, or swelling Cough or shortness of breath Diarrhea	Sore throat Shaking chills Weakness and easy fatigability Dyspnea on exertion Burning during urination Nasal congestion

Dental Management

The WBC status of patients with a suspicious clinical presentation should be evaluated with a CBC and differential. Consultation with the patient's physician is often appropriate with abnormal WBCs.

Although no clear evidence is present in the literature, the use of prophylactic antibiotics before and after invasive dental procedures seems prudent for an ANC < 500 to 1,000/μL. This recommendation is related to the mouth as a common source of bacteremia, although the presence of poor oral health may place a patient at greater risk of bacteremia than infrequent invasive dental procedures.

LEUKOCYTOSIS (increase in WBC)

Similar to a deficient WBC, an elevated WBC can be associated with numerous etiologies. The presence

TABLE 5–11: Selected Examples of Etiology of Leukocytosis	
Etiology	*Examples*
Neutrophilia (↑ neutrophils)	
Reactive causes	Infection; Inflammation; Tissue damage; Metabolic disorders; Steroid therapy; Growth factor therapy; Splenectomy
Underlying medical conditions/malignancy	Polycythemia vera; Myelogenous leukemia
Lymphocytosis (↑ lymphocytes)	
Infectious disease	Viral; Bacterial
Other reactive	Allergy; Autoimmune disease; Hyperthyroidism; Malnutrition; Drug reaction
Malignant conditions	Lymphocytic leukemia; Lymphoma; Mycosis fungoides; Plasma cell leukemia

of a leukocytosis is most often related to an increased neutrophil (neutrophilia) and/or lymphocyte (lymphocytosis) count, both of which may be related to a reactive or malignant etiology. An increase in the WBC will not by itself lead to specific signs and symptoms unless a malignancy is the underlying etiology. Pallor, weakness, and fatigue may be presenting signs and symptoms of leukemia. In most cases, the etiology of the leukocytosis is an underlying disease, such as a bacterial infection. Treatment of such cases involves resolution of the underlying microbial infection.

LEUKEMIA

Dramatic leukocytosis is seen in leukemia, characterized by an elevated percentage of immature white blood cells (blasts) in the peripheral circulation. As stated previously, constitutional symptoms that occur in leukemia include nausea, fever, weight loss, fatigue, hemoptysis, epistaxis, and malaise. The disorder can affect any age group but is more prevalent over the age of 40 years. 13.5 per 100 000 new cases of leukemia are diagnosed per year. Approximately 1.5% of men and women will be diagnosed with leukemia at some point during their lifetime.

Four major categories of leukemia are recognized: acute lymphocytic leukemia (ALL), acute myelogenous leukemia (AML), chronic lymphocytic leukemia, (CLL), and chronic myelogenous leukemia (CML). The most common type of leukemia in adults is AML, whereas ALL is more prevalent in children. The etiology of leukemia can be genetic, environmental, a late effect of exposure to ionizing radiation, or idiopathic. Leukemia is treated with toxic chemotherapy, stem cell transplantation including autologous (self) hema-topoietic stem cell transplantation targeted immune therapy (e.g., monoclonal antibodies) and radiation therapy.

Oral Manifestations

A patient presenting with clinical signs of an oral infection (e.g., swelling, purulence, pain, and erythema) may also have an elevated WBC. Leukemic patients with extremely high WBCs (e.g., 100,000/µL) rarely present with a chloroma (nontender nodules composed of granulocytes). Intraoral extramedullary leukemic infiltrates have been reported. Mucositis affects the vast majority of patients treated for leukemia. Mucositis resulting from chemotherapy toxicity can be a treatment-limiting complication in patients treated for the disease.

TABLE 5–12: Oral Health Care Considerations In Leukemia
Before treatment
Comprehensive history, examination
Prechemotherapy clearance, evaluation pretransplantation
Clear or eliminate possible sites of infection
During treatment
Follow mucositis/opportunistic infections
Treat dental infections aggressively
Home care education
After treatment
Frequent dental recall in remission
Monitor for signs of disease

Dental Management

Pretreatment evaluation and assessment should be completed with the goal of eliminating all potential sources of oral infection, which may complicate chemotherapy. Consultation with the patient's oncologist prior to the initiation of chemotherapy is necessary to determine the specific diagnosis, prognosis and anticipated mode of treatment. When extractions are indicated, they should be completed 10 to 14 days prior to the initiating chemotherapy. The clinician should be aware of the possible appearance of intraoral extramedullary leukemic infiltrates, which can mimic periodontal pathology.

A patient presenting with an oral infection and an elevated WBC requires appropriate dental management to include the following: removal of the dental source of infection by root canal therapy or extraction, appropriate antibiotic therapy (for example, penicillin VK 500 mg qid X 7 days or clindamycin 300 mg qid X 7 days), and follow-up to ensure resolution of infection. Patients on chemotherapy for leukemia should have their white blood cell and platelet counts monitored closely to prevent complications from dental interventions. Antibiotic prophylaxis may be recommended for patients with ANC < 1000 µL. Neutropenic patients may develop an aggressive infection and oral ulcerations with minimal signs of localized inflammation.

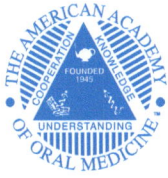

6 Immunology and Infectious Diseases

HIV/AIDS

EPIDEMIOLOGY

Human immunodeficiency virus (HIV), the causative agent of acquired immune deficiency syndrome (AIDS), was first identified in 1983; however, the first documented cases of AIDS, reported in 1981 by the Centers for Disease Control and Prevention (CDC), marked the beginning of an epidemic. According to CDC, there were about 36.7 million people were living with HIV worldwide and 1.8 million of new cases of HIV in 2016. The CDC indicates that about 1.1 million people in USA were living with HIV at the end of 2015 and of those people, about 15 % or 1 in 7, did not know they were infected. According to CDC, among adults and adolescents living with HIV in 2014; 62% received some HIV medical care; only 48% were retained in continuous HIV care and 49% had achieved viral suppression. In 2016, the annual number of HIV diagnoses declined 5% between 2011 and 2015. This has led to a significant shift in public policy, with the CDC now recommending that all individuals aged 13 to 64 years have HIV tests as part of routine medical care. This is an important strategy to reduce the spread of HIV since young individuals aged 13-24 are especially affected by HIV. In 2015, they comprised 16% of the US population but accounted for 22% of all new HIV diagnoses.

The epidemic is growing most rapidly among minority populations, with CDC data indicating that, in 2016, 44% of HIV diagnoses are African Americans and 69% (AA and Hispanics/Latinos) of all new HIV diagnoses occurred in minority Americans. From 2011 to 2015, diagnoses among all women declined 16%; among all heterosexuals, diagnoses declined 15% and among people who inject drugs (PWID), diagnoses declined 17%. Successful implementation of rapid testing and appropriate use of antiretroviral medications during labor and delivery have significantly decreased maternal child transmission in the United States. According to CDC, between 1994 and 2010, an estimated 21,956 cases of perinatally acquired HIV infections were prevented.

PATHOGENESIS

HIV, a retrovirus, is found in blood, semen, vaginal fluid, breast milk, saliva, and tears. Spread of HIV occurs through sexual contact with an infected person or sharing needles with someone who is infected. The spread of HIV via infected blood transfusions or blood clotting factors has been virtually eliminated in the United States since the routine screening of all blood products.

HIV targets cells with a surface molecule called cluster designation 4 (CD4), which are found on CD4+ T lymphocytes, blood monocytes, tissue macrophages, natural killer cells, dendritic cells, hematopoietic stem cells, endothelial cells, microglial cells in the brain, and gastrointestinal epithelial cells. HIV replicates inside cells using the reverse transcriptase enzyme to convert their ribonucleic acid (RNA) into deoxyribonucleic acid (DNA) prior to incorporation into the host cell's genes; the infected cells can then release virions by surface budding. Death of the CD4 T cells occurs via direct cell killing as the budding virus disrupts the cell membrane, syncytia formation or fusion of infected to non-infected cells, and programmed cell death or apoptosis.

Primary HIV infection is associated with high levels of HIV viral load and an initial decrease in the absolute CD4+ T-cell count. Production of antibodies and activation of CD8+ T cells signal the progression into a clinically latent period. During this period, levels of HIV viral load remain low, although HIV viral replication continues, with a resultant slow decline in immune function. The final phase of HIV infection occurs when a significant number of CD4 lymphocytes have been destroyed and when production of new ones cannot match the rate of cell loss.

Physical Evaluation

Successful medical care for HIV-positive individuals includes early detection of the infection and appropriate referral for care. Many of the conditions that put immunocompromised patients at risk for disease can be detected early, by means of a thorough history and physical evaluation.

Initial evaluation of the patient includes the following:

- A comprehensive physical examination, focusing on subjective findings elicited in the history
- Review of systems
- Baseline/intake laboratory work (CD4+ T-cell count, plasma HIV RNA load, drug-resistance testing, complete blood count (CBC) with differential and platelets, chemistry profile (electrolytes, creatinine, blood urea nitrogen, liver transaminases), lipid profile (total cholesterol, low-density lipoprotein, high density lipoprotein, triglycerides), glucose, hepatitis screening, purified protein derivative testing
- Perform immunizations for pneumonia (Pneumovax) and influenza (as appropriate) and other immunizations as indicated
- Referral to social services, mental health, community, and other clinic services as needed

Follow-up visits every 3 months are recommended to conduct a full physical examination, evaluate new symptoms, update laboratory values, check adherence and response to HIV medications and medications for other conditions, discuss risk reduction, and monitor compliance with other services.

Disease Staging

HIV disease staging and classification systems provide clinicians with important information about HIV disease stage and clinical management. Two major classification systems are currently in use: the CDC classification system (Table 6-1) and the World Health Organization (WHO) Clinical Staging and Disease Classification System. The CDC disease staging system was revised in 2014 to adapt to the recent changes in diagnostic criteria. This classification includes four stages (0, 1, 2, 3 or unknown). The staging is based primarily on CD4+ T-lymphocyte count, whereas the WHO Clinical Staging and Disease Classification System (revised in 2005) classifies HIV disease on the basis of symptoms and clinical manifestations.

Medical Management

The cornerstone of successful medical management of the HIV-positive patient involves suppression of HIV replication and prophylaxis of opportunistic infections associated with diminishing immune function with appropriate medications. The goal of antiretroviral therapy (ART) is the durable suppression of HIV replication, and the potent combination antiretroviral therapy, consisting of 3 or more of the 25 antiretroviral drugs currently available. This approach has greatly improved the health and survival rates of HIV-infected patients. Drug resistance profiles (genotype, phenotype, or both) are recommended prior to initiation of ART owing to the estimated prevalence of ART drug resistance in 6 to 16% of treatment-naive patients. In fact, approximately 10% to 17% of ART-naive individuals have resistance mutations to at least one ARV drug. Up to 8%, but generally less than 5%, of transmitted viruses will exhibit resistance to drugs from more than 1 class. The failure of an ART regimen when

	Age on date of CD4+ T-lymphocyte test					
Stage	**<1 yr**		**1–5 yrs**		**≥6 yrs**	
	Cells/µL	**%**	**Cells/µL**	**%**	**Cells/µL**	**%**
1	≥ 1,500	≥ 34	≥ 1,000	≥ 30	≥ 500	≥ 26
2	750–1,499	26–33	500–999	22–29	200–499	14–25
3	<750	<26	<500	<22	<200	<14

TABLE 6-1: HIV infection stage* based on age-specific CD4+ T-lymphocyte count or CD4+ T-lymphocyte percentage of total lymphocytes

* The stage is based primarily on the CD4+ T-lymphocyte count; the CD4+ T-lymphocyte count takes precedence over the CD4 T-lymphocyte percentage, and the percentage is considered only if the count is missing. There are three situations in which the stage is not based on this table: 1) if the criteria for stage 0 are met, the stage is 0 regardless of criteria for other stages (CD4 T-lymphocyte test results and opportunistic illness diagnoses); 2) if the criteria for stage 0 are not met and a stage-3-defining opportunistic illness has been diagnosed (Appendix), then the stage is 3 regardless of CD4 T-lymphocyte test results; or 3) if the criteria for stage 0 are not met and information on the above criteria for other stages is missing, then the stage is classified as unknown.

Used with permission of the CDC.gov

accompanied by drug resistance usually means that subsequent regimens are less likely to succeed.

The absolute CD4+ cell count (primarily) and CD4+ percentage (if CD4+ count is missing) are used for disease staging and to determine when to start ART and prophylaxis against opportunistic infections. The HIV RNA level (viral load), when used in conjunction with the CD4 count, also provides prognostic information in patients who are naive to ART. Data from various cohort studies have demonstrated the strong relationship between a lower CD4 count or higher viral load and the risk of progression to AIDS:

ART is recommended for all individuals with HIV, regardless of CD4 cell count, to reduce the morbidity and mortality associated with HIV infection (AI). ART is also recommended for individuals with HIV to prevent HIV transmission. While ART is recommended for all patients, the following conditions increase the urgency to initiate therapy:

- Pregnancy (refer to the Perinatal Guidelines for more detailed recommendations on the management of pregnant women with HIV)
- AIDS-defining conditions, including HIV-associated dementia (HAD) and AIDS-associated malignancies
- Acute opportunistic infections
- Lower CD4 counts (<200cells/mm^3)
- HIV-associated nephropathy (HIVAN)
- Acute/early infection
- HIV/Hepatitis B virus coinfection
- HIV/Hepatitis C virus coinfection

Patient adherence is critical to the success of a particular regimen; however, the side effects of ART are many and varied (Table 6-2), making adherence difficult. In addition, the side effects may impact the delivery of dental care.

Laboratory Values

The CD4-lymphocyte count is a measure of both immunocompetence and disease progression (see Table 6-4). HIV viral load measurements predict the rate of disease progression and is an important treatment response to ART.

TABLE 6–2: Side Effects of HAART	
Drug Category	**Most Common Side Effects**
Nucleoside and nucleotide reverse transcriptase inhibitors	Headache, malaise, nausea, vomiting and diarrhea, peripheral neuropathy
Non-nucleoside reverse transcriptase inhibitors	Rash, central nervous system symptoms(dizziness, somnolence, insomnia, abnormal dreams, confusion, impaired thinking), increased liver function tests in patients with previous history of hepatitis B and/or C
Protease inhibitors	Hyperlipidemia, hyperglycemia, fat redistribution, circumoral paresthesia, hepatitis
Coformulations (multiple active components)	Bone marrow suppression, nausea, headache, possible nephropathy, hepatitis
Fusion blocker	Injection-site reactions: erythema, induration, pain/tenderness

TABLE 6–3: Prophylaxis of Opportunistic Infections		
Disease Process	**Medications**	**CD4+ T Cells/µL**
Pneumocystis carinii pneumonia	Bactrim; Dapsone; Atovaquone	CD4 < 200 200 – 300 with HIV viral load > 100,000/mL, symptomatic HIV
Toxoplasma gondii	Bactrim; Dapsone + pyrimethamine	50 – 100 cells
Mycobacterium avium complex	Azithromycin; Clarithromycin; Rifabutin	50 – 100 cells
Cytomegalovirus	Ganciclovir; Valganciclovir, foscarnet, cidofovir	50 – 100 cells
Cryptosporidiosis	initiate or optimize ART for immune restoration to CD4 count >100 cells/µL	<100cells/uL
Microsporidiosis	initiate or optimize ART for immune restoration to CD4 count >100 cells/µL	<100cells/uL
Mycobacterium tuberculosis infection and disease	isoniazid, pyridoxine, rifampin, rifabutin, rifapentine, pyrazinamide, ethambutol, moxifloxacin, levofloxacin, nevirapine	any CD4 cell count

TABLE 6 – 3: Prophylaxis of Opportunistic Infections (continued)		
Disease Process	*Medications*	*CD4+ T Cells/µL*
Bacterial respiratory disease	beta-lactam (ceftriaxone, cefotaxime, ampicillin-sulbactam), azithromycin, clarithromycin, amoxicillin, amoxicillin/clavulanate, cefpodoxime, cefuroxime, levofloxacin, moxifloxacin, doxyclycline	any CD4 cell count
Bacterial enteric infection	ciprofloxacin, ceftriaxone, cefotaxime, levofloxacin, moxifloxacin, trimethoprim, azithromycin, vancomycin	<200 CD4 cell count
Bartonellosis	doxycycline, erythromycin, rifampin, gentamicin, azithromycin, clarithromycin	< 50 cells/mm³
Syphilis	benzathine penicillin G, doxycycline, ceftriaxone azithromycin	transient decrease in CD4
Mucocutaneous candidiasis	fluconazole, clotrimazole troches, miconazole, itraconazole, posaconazole, nystatin, voriconazole, isavuconazole, caspofungin, micafungin, anidulafungin, amphotericin B deoxycholate, lipid formulation of amphotericin B	< 200 cells/mm³
▪ *Invasive mycoses*		
cryptococcosis	flucytosine, amphotericin B, fluconazole, itraconazole	<100 cells/uL
histoplasmosis	itraconazole, amphotericin B, itraconazole, posaconazole, voriconazole	<150 cells/uL
coccidioidomycosis	fluconazole, itraconazole, voriconazole, posaconazole, amphotericin B	<250 cells/uL
Herpes simplex virus	valacyclovir, famciclovir, acyclovir	common; <250 cells/uL
VZV	valacyclovir, famciclovir, acyclovir, ganciclovir, foscarnet	<200 cells/uL
HH8	optimization of ART, valaganciclovir, ganciclovir, rituximab	<200 cells/uL
HPV	imiquimod 5% cream, sinecatechins 15% ointment	low count
Hepatitis B virus	emtricitabine, interferon, immunoglobulin, tenofovir alafenamide, tenofovir disoproxile fumarate	<200 cells/uL
▪ *Geographically associated opportunistic infection of specific consideration*		
malaria	trimethoprim-sulfamethoxazole	<350 cells/uL
penicilliosis marneffei	itraconazole, fluconazole, amphotericin B, voriconazole	<100 cells/uL
leishmaniasis	amphotericin B, pentavalent antimony	<200 cells/uL
Chagas disease	benznidazole, niturtimox	<200 cells/uL
isosporiasis (cystoisosporiasis)	pirimethamine, ciprofloxacin, trimethoprim, sulfamethoxazole	<200 cells/uL

A higher viral load equals a higher rate of viral replication; it causes a more rapid decline in CD4 count, more rapid disease progression, and resistance to ART. Regardless of the CD4 count, an increase in viral load results in a significant decrease in AIDS-free survival.

Dental Management
Access to dental services remains a major unmet need for people living with HIV/AIDS; however, the dental team plays two significant roles in the management of the HIV-positive patient:

TABLE 6–4: CD-4 Count and Viral Load Progression of HIV			
CD4 Count	**Viral Load**	**AIDS Progression in Men (%)**	
(cells/µL)	**(copies/mL)**	**Over 3 yr**	**Over 9 yr**
< 200	< 10,000	14	64
	10,000–30,000	50	90
	> 30,000	86	100
200–349	< 10,000	7	66
	10,000–30,000	36	85
	> 30,000	64	93
> 350	< 10,000	7	54
	10,000–30,000	15	74
	> 30,000	40	85

Adapted from Mellors JW, Rinaldo CR Jr, Gupta P, et al. Prognosis in HIV-1 infection predicted by the quantity of virus in plasma. Science 1996;272:1167–70.

- *The provision of oral health services.* The main concern when providing dental treatment to HIV-positive patients is the presence of neutropenia or thrombocytopenia; however, there are no significant differences in postoperative complications between HIV-positive and -negative patients, regardless of the severity of the immunosuppression. The provision of dental care to HIV-positive patients depends more on the patient's sense of "well-being" and ability to pay for services.

- *The diagnosis and management of oral lesions.* Since the advent of combination ART, the prevalence of HIV-related oral lesions has declined; however, the oral cavity is still one of the most common areas of symptoms in patients with HIV infection. The occurrence of oral lesions is strongly indicative of changes in immune status (CD4 cell count and HIV viral load) and requires referral of the patient to their primary health care provider for evaluation of immune

TABLE 6–5: Oral Manifestations of HIV			
Condition	**Clinical Appearance**	**CD4 Cell Count**	**Diagnosis**
Erythematous candidiasis	Red atrophic patches on tongue and palate	≤ 400 cells/µL	Clinical appearance
Pseudomembranous candidiasis	White curd-like lesions throughout oral cavity	≤ 200 cells/µL	KOH stain Culture
Herpes simplex	Ulcers on keratinized tissue that tend to persist longer in individuals with significant immunosuppression; an extensive, deep non healing ulcerations from HSV were reported in profoundly immunocompromised patient with CD4 counts of <100c/uL	Can occur at any CD4 cell count	Cytology Culture
Kaposi sarcoma	Red, blue, or purplish lesions that are flat or nodular and solitary or multiple; lesions appear most commonly on the hard palate but also occur on gingival surfaces and elsewhere in the mouth (KS and primary effusion lymphoma frequently occurred in advanced immunosuppressed HIV infected patients and lesions are non tender)	Can occur at any CD4 cell count (CD4 < 200 cells/ul)	Biopsy and histologic examination Dx – cytologic and immunologic cell markers and histology
Hairy leukoplakia	Asymptomatic striated white "hairy" lesions on lateral border of the tongue	≤ 400 cells/µL	Biopsy and histologic examination
Major aphthous	Large ulcers on nonkeratinized tissue	< 100 cells/µL	Biopsy and histologic examination
Oral warts human papilloma infection)	Painless solitary or multiple nodules with smooth or cauliflower-like surface	Can occur at any CD4 cell count	Clinical appearance Biopsy human papillomavirus typing
Necrotizing ulcerative periodontitis	Ulcerative lesions of the periodontium with rapidly progressive loss of underlying bone	< 100 cells/µL	Clinical appearance

status. Factors associated with the occurrence of oral lesions include CD4 T-cell counts < 200/μL, HIV viral load greater than 3,000 copies/mL, xerostomia, poor oral hygiene, and smoking (see Table 6-5).

Prior to provision of dental services
- Obtain a thorough medical history, review of systems, and social history
- Obtain CBC with differential for invasive procedures
- Obtain prothrombin time/partial thromboplastin time or international normalized ratio in patients with a history of elevated liver function tests prior to surgical procedures
- Regardless of CD4+ cell count, infective endocarditis IE prophylaxis is NOT required unless
  1. The patient has a cardiac condition requiring IE prophylaxis according to the guidelines set by the American Heart Association
  2. The patient has an absolute neutrophil count of < 500 cells/mm³ and invasive dental procedures are planned.

Timely management of oral pain is necessary to support adherence to ART and maintain adequate nutritional intake.

Diagnosis and Management of Oral Lesions
In patients with unknown HIV status, oral lesions may be the first indication of HIV disease. The presence of an oral lesion in an HIV-positive patient on ART may indicate treatment failure.

AUTOIMMUNE DISORDERS
Autoimmune disorders are a frequent cause of dental morbidity owing to the skeletal and oral complications that arise from specific diseases and from dental sequelae occurring secondary to medical treatment. The following summary describes two autoimmune conditions that may present in dental practice, regardless of specialty.

RHEUMATOID ARTHRITIS
Definition
Rheumatoid arthritis (RA) is a chronic systemic inflammatory disease that primarily affects the synovium of joints. The synovial tissues in RA proliferate uncontrollably, consequently resulting in excess fluid accumulation and erosive destruction of bone, cartilage, tendon, and ligament. RA can be debilitating, particularly in advanced stages, and result in a compromised quality of life and potential mortality. The etiology of RA is likely multiple and yet to be determined. It is established that genetics may increase the risk for the development of RA and the severity of the disease. It has been suggested that bacteria such as *Mycobacteria*, *Streptococcus*, *Mycoplasma*, *Escherichia coli*, and *Helicobacter pylori*; viruses such as rubella, Epstein-Barr virus, and parvovirus; and superantigens may be triggers for RA. In addition, infectious triggers resulting in arthritic syndromes such as rheumatic

Table 6–6: Clinical Presentation of RA
Arthralgia
Swelling
Warmth
Morning stiffness
Fatigue
Anorexia
Weight loss
Low-grade fever
Joint held in flexion
Radial deviation
Pain with mobility
Subtle onset
Worse after prolonged rest
Warmth and activity improve symptoms

TABLE 6–7: Articular Involvement of RA
Hand and wrist: proximal interphalangeal and metacarpo-phalangeal; radial deviation
Ankle and foot: tenderness, swelling, and possible subluxation of metatarsophalangeal
Large joints (shoulders, hips): symmetric between sides and within individual joints
Knee: popliteal cysts
Neck: C1–C2 subluxation and compression
Temporomandibular joints: involved 50–75% of the time in rheumatoid arthritis

TABLE 6–8: Extra Articular Involvement in RA
Skin: subcutaneous nodules 25% of the time in seropositive RA; extensor surface common
Cardiac: uncommon pericardial perfusion
Pulmonary: pleural effusion, rheumatoid nodules, parenchymal lung disease, and interstitial fibrosis
Eye: keroconjunctivitis sicca from secondary Sjögren's syndrome, scleritis
Neurologic: peripheral neuropathy, nerve entrapment (carpal tunnel syndrome)
Hematologic: thrombocytosis, anemia
Felty syndrome: triad of RA, splenomegaly, and neutropenia
RA = rheumatoid arthritis.

fever, reactive arthritis (Reiter syndrome), and Lyme arthritis have been implicated. It is likely that the etiology of RA is multifactorial and involves the complex interaction between genetic and environmental factors and the immune system of synovial joints.

The prevalence of RA is range from 0.41% to 0.52% in USA from 2004–2014 among adults, and prevalence among females was more than twice the prevalence among males Onset for RA is typically 45 years in men but can occur at any age. Among women, the peak onset is 45 years, and the risk of developing RA plateaus. The incidence of RA varies with age and is approximately 20 in 100,000 for men and approximately 40 in 100,000 for women. RA is a lifelong disease, and its prevalence increases with each decade.

Physical Evaluation/Status

All synovial (diarthroidal) joints can be affected by RA. Joint involvement begins with the small joints of the hand, followed by the wrists, knees, elbows, ankles, hips, and shoulders. Occasionally, the temporomandibular, crico-arytenoid, sternoclavicular, and C1–C2 spine joints are involved, as well as an increased risk for osteoporosis in advanced RA. RA does not affect the distal interphalangeal and small joints of the toe (see Tables 6-6, 6-7, and 6-8).

Diagnosis

There is no single finding in the history and examination or laboratory test that is pathognomonic of RA. RA is diagnosed based on the American College of Rheumatology criteria (revised 2010) outlined in Tables 6-9, 6-10, and 6-11.

Laboratory

No specific laboratory test is pathognomonic of RA.

Medical Treatment

The primary goal for RA treatment is early aggressive treatment that encourages disease-continued suppression. This includes medications, especially disease modifying anti-rheumatic drugs, range of motion exercises, joint protection, and assistive devices. Surgical options are considered in the event of severe mechanical symptoms and include arthroplasty, synovectomy, and prosthetic joint replacement.

TABLE 6–9: Classification Criteria for Rheumatoid Arthritis*	Score
Target population (Who should be tested?): Patients who	
1) have at least 1 joint with definite clinical synovitis (swelling)*	
2) with the synovitis not better explained by another disease †	
Classification criteria for RA (score-based algorithm: add score of categories A-D; a score of ≥ 6/10 is needed for classification of a patient as having definitive RA) ‡	
A. Joint involvement §	
1 large joint¶	0
2–10 large joints	1
1–3 small joints (with or without involvement of large joints) #	2
4–10 small joints (with or without involvement of large joints)	3
> 10 joints (at least 1 small joint) **	5
B. Serology (at least 1 test result is needed for classification † †	
Negative RF *and* negative ACPA	0
Low-positive RF *or* low-positive ACPA	2
High-positive RF *or* high-positive ACPA	3
C. Acute-phase reactants (at least 1 test result is needed for classification) ‡ ‡	
Normal CRP *and* normal ESR	0
Abnormal CRP *or* abnormal ESR	1
D. Duration of symptoms §§	
< 6 weeks	0
≥ 6 weeks	1

* Used with permission of the CDC.gov [from the The 2010 American College of Rheumatology/European League Against Rheumatism classification criteria for rheumatoid arthritis]

Dental Management

The dental management for patients with rheumatoid disease is outlined in Table 6-13 on the following page.

TABLE 6−10: Characteristics of Rheumatoid Arthritis

Serum rheumatoid factor: present in approximately 80% of patients

Anemia: present in 80% of RA; proportional to activity of the disease

Thrombocytosis ESR and CRP levels: present in 90% of RA patients; elevated levels indicative of poor prognosis

Antinuclear antibodies: positive in 30% of RA patients

Synovial fluid analysis: WBC count 5,000–100,000/mm3

CRP = C-reactive protein; ESR = erythrocyte sedimentation rate; RA = rheumatoid arthritis; WBC = white blood cell.

TABLE 6−11: Imaging of RA

Conventional radiograph: Joints: cysts, erosion, osteopenia, joint space narrowing, calcifications, separations and fractures

Cervical spine: inflammation and destruction of C1–C2 cartilage, bone, and ligaments

MRI and CT: supplement conventional radiography; for more detailed soft tissue and bony involvement visualization

CT = computed tomography; MRI = magnetic resonance imaging.

SYSTEMIC LUPUS ERYTHEMATOSUS

Lupus erythematosus presents in two forms: (1) discoid lupus erythematosus (DLE), which predominantly affects the skin, and (2) systemic lupus erythematosus (SLE), a more generalized disease affecting multiple organs. DLE presents as benign, chronic, erythematous scaly plaques of the face, scalp, and ears. This guideline focuses on SLE (see Table 6 –15).

SLE is an autoimmune disease with multiple presentations and may include fever, rash, hair loss, arthritis, pleuritis, pericarditis, nephritis, anemia, leukopenia, thrombocytopenia, and central nervous system disease. SLE can have periods of remission and acute or chronic recurrences. The etiology of SLE remains elusive. It is an autoimmune disease based on a polyclonal B-cell inflammatory response affecting the connective tissue of blood vessels, joints, kidney, and serous surfaces, among others. Pathogenic antibody production as a reaction to antigens forms immune complexes that deposit in various organs and tissues, causing inflammation and vasculopathy. SLE can occur at any age but predominantly occurs in females (15:1), with peak incidence between the ages of 15 and 40 years. The prevalence of SLE is between 40 and 50 cases per 100,000 population and highest among Asians in Hawaii, blacks, and certain Native Americans.

TABLE 6−12: Pharmacologic Treatments of RA

Drug Category	Drug	Mode of Action
DMARDs* (nonbiologic)	Sulfasalazine Hydroxychloroquine Azathioprine Leflunomide	Reduce disease activity and/or prevent joint damage See individual drugs for side effects and toxicity
	Methotrexate	Immunosuppressive and anti-inflammatory effects
DMARDs* (biologic)	TNF –alpha blocker	Target cytokines or their receptors
	Etanercept	
	Infliximab	
	Rituximab	Monoclonal antibody
NSAIDs and aspirin		Anti-inflammatory and pain relief effects Caution: gastrointestinal bleeding and ulcerations; nephrotoxicity, hepatotoxicity
COX-2 inhibitor	Celecoxib	Anti-inflammatory and pain relief effect Increased risk of cardiovascular events
Glucocorticoids	Prednisone	Immunosuppressive and anti-inflammatory effects Caution: hyperglycemia, edema, infections, peptic ulcers, myopathy, hypokalemia

COX = cyclooxygenase; DMARD = disease-modifying antirheumatic drug; NSAID = nonsteroidal anti-inflammatory drug.
*Many of the above-mentioned medications have serious side effects.

TABLE 6–13: Dental Management of RA	
Therapy	*Considerations*
NSAIDs for dental pain and TMD	Check patient's current medications, especially use of other methotrexate and NSAIDs Consider use of GI-protective agents such as misoprostol
Folic acid	Treatment of stomatitis secondary to methotrexate
Replacement therapy for adrenal suppression	Prevent cardiovascular collapse secondary to glucocorticoid use
Intravenous/intramuscular hydrocortisone	Check for blood pressure drops secondary to glucocorticoid use
Long-lasting local anesthesia (bupivacaine) and sedative	For surgical stress in adrenally suppressed (individuals secondary to glucocorticoid use)
Administer antibiotic prophylaxis	For temporomandibular joint replacement surgery For immunosuppression apparent
Soft diet restriction	TMJ dysfunction
Physical therapy	Improve jaw function
Hemostasis considerations	Felty syndrome (may result in thrombocytopenia)
Oral hygiene and dietary instruction, fluoride therapy, chlorhexidine therapy, xerostomia treatment, periodic radiographs, conservative treatment plans, and frequent recalls	Secondary Sjogren's syndrome
Pilocarpine hydrochloride	Dry mouth
Comfortable dental chair, including pillow use, short appointments	Depending on severity of RA
Specially designed toothbrush, electric toothbrush, floss holders, irrigating devices, chlorhexidine, fluoride rinses	Severe RA affecting dexterity
GI = gastrointestinal; NSAID = nonsteroidal anti-inflammatory drug; RA = rheumatoid arthritis; TMD = temporomandibular joint disorder; TMJ = temporomandibular joint.	

TABLE 6–14: Considerations for Oral Conditions
Stomatitis secondary to methotrexate, gold, d-penicillamine, and NSAID use
TMJ dysfunction secondary to granulomatous involvement of articular surfaces
Periodontal disease, including loss of alveolar bone and teeth owing to poor oral hygiene secondary to functional impairment
Chronic xerostomia resulting in difficulty swallowing, speaking, intolerance to spicy foods, oral candidiasis, and secondary caries
NSAID = nonsteroidal anti-inflammatory drug; TMJ = temporomandibular joint.

Physical Evaluation

The American College of Rheumatology criteria for classification of SLE are based on the presence of any 4 or more of the 11 criteria being present (Table 6-17).

Medical Treatment

There is no cure for SLE. However, there are measures that can be adopted to manage the signs and symptoms of SLE (Table 6-18).

Dental Management

The dental management for patients with SLE is outlined in Table 6-19.

Oral manifestations for patients with SLE are outlined in Table 6-20.

ORGAN TRANSPLANTATION

Transplantation has become the treatment of choice for the restoration of function and preservation of life in end-stage

TABLE 6–15: Features of SLE	
Features	**Presentation**
General	Fatigue, malaise, fever, weight loss, arthralgia/myalgia
Skin	Butterfly rash, discoid LE cells, photosensitivity, mucous ulcers, alopecia, purpura, Raynaud phenomenon, urticaria
Renal	Nephrosis
Pulmonary	Pleurisy, effusions, pneumonia
Cardiac	Pericarditis, murmurs, electrocardiographic changes
CNS	Functional, psychosis, seizures
Others	Gastrointestinal, lymphadenopathy, splenomegaly, hepatomegaly, hematologic
CNS = central nervous system; LE = lupus erythematosus.	

TABLE 6–17: Manifestations of SLE

1. Malar rash: butterfly rash
2. Discoid rash
3. Photosensitivity: skin rash secondary to light sensitivity
4. Oral ulcers
5. Arthritis: multiple joint involvement characterized by noneroded bone, tenderness, swelling, effusion
6. Serositis: pleuritis, pericarditis
7. Renal disorder: persistent proteinuria and cellular casts
8. Neurologic disorder: seizures and psychosis
9. Hematologic disorder: hemolytic anemia, leukopenia, lymphopenia, thrombocytopenia
10. Immunologic disorder: see Table 6-16
11. Antinuclear antibody: abnormal titer of antinuclear antibody by immunofluorescence

TABLE 6–16: Imaging, Laboratory, and Special Tests for SLE	
Study	**Finding**
Antinuclear antibody	Positive in 95% of patients
Other autoantibodies	Anti-dsDNA assay: elevated in 65–80% Rheumatoid factor: positive in 20% Antigen to Smith (Sm) antigen: positive in 10–25% Antibodies to Ro SS-A antigen: positive in 15–20% Antibodies to La (SS-B) antigen: positive in 5–20%
CBC with differential	Hemolytic anemia, leukopenia, lymphopenia, thrombocytopenia
Renal function	Creatinine and blood urine nitrogen
Urinalysis	Protein and casts
ESR, PTT, anticardiolipin antibodies	Patients with history of thromboembolic events
Biopsy: skin or oral mucosa	Collagenous and fibrinoid changes, cellular necrosis, granulomatous reactions, and periarterial sclerosis
Others	Chest radiography and pulmonary function tests: investigate pulmonary involvement Echocardiogram: history of heart disease
CBC = complete blood count; DNA = deoxyribonucleic acid; ESR = erythrocyte sedimentation rate; PTT = partial thromboplastin time.	

organ disease. Innovative surgical techniques have played a major role in enhancing the success of organ transplants, leading to improved graft and patient survival. Advances in the biology of organ preservation and insights into the biology of immune responses to transplanted tissues have resulted in improved patient outcomes. The development of immunosuppressive agents to prevent rejection of the transplants while minimizing the morbidities continues to be studied.

In 2018, 114,000 patients were on the national transplant waiting list. In 2017, more than 34,500 transplants were performed.

Virtually all types of solid organs and tissues have been transplanted, whereas hematopoietic cell transplants (HCTs) have been used to treat various hematologic and some nonhematologic malignancies and disorders.

TABLE 6–18: Medical Management of SLE	
Treatment	**Management**
Nonpharmacologic	Avoid sun exposure and use high ultraviolet factor sunscreen Monitor exacerbations; obtain laboratory data and frequent follow-ups for chronic SLE
Pharmacologic	Aspirin and NSAIDs for mild SLE Antimalarials for dermatologic disease Glucocorticoids and cytotoxic agents for severe SLE Antipsychotics and anticonvulsants for CNS symptoms Vincristine and immunoglobulins for thrombocytopenia Biological agents

CNS = central nervous system; NSAID = nonsteroidal anti-inflammatory drug; SLE = systemic lupus erythematosus.

TABLE 6–19: Dental Manaegement of SLE

1. Determine the basis for SLE diagnosis, including onset, duration, and severity; associated organ involvement; current and past treatments; consult and coordinate with patient's primary care physician, dermatologist, rheumatologist, and other health care providers prior to performing dental treatment to determine patient's status and stability

2. Determine patient's laboratory results, including CBC with differential, PT, PTT, and BT, to monitor normochromic normocytic anemia, hemolytic anemia, leukopenia, thrombocytopenia and hemostasis; creatinine clearance, serum creatinine, and BUN if renal disease present

3. Caution with performing elective dental procedures, especially in patients with a history of post-surgery SLE flare-ups

4. Assess risk for adrenal suppression and insufficiency if corticosteroid medication is being used

5. Pre- and postsurgical antibiotic for patients taking cytotoxic and immunosuppressive drugs with an increased risk of infection

6. Consider use of antibiotic prophylaxis in patients with increased risk for infective endocarditis secondary to cardiac complications

BUN = blood urea nitrogen; BT = bleeding time; CBC = complete blood count; PT = prothrombin time; PTT = partial thromboplastin time; SLE = systemic lupus erythematosus.

TABLE 6–20: Oral Manifestations of SLE	
Oral ulcers	Lip and mucosa involved in 5–25% of patients Mucosa: possibly painful, nonspecific, erythematous with white spots and radiating lines (resemble lichen planus or leukoplakia) Lip: silvery, scaly margin; occurs with exposure to sun Also screen for angular cheilitis, mucositis, and glossitis
Xerostomia	May result in rampant caries and candidiasis More severe in patients taking corticosteroids and immunosuppressive drugs
Temporomandibular disorders	Pain and compromised jaw function

TABLE 6–21: Types of Transplants		
Type of Transplantation		
Type of Graft	**Procedure**	**Description**
Autograft	Autologous	Transplant from self
Isograft	Syngeneic	Transplant between genetically identical individuals (monozygotic twin)
Allograft	Allogeneic	Transplant from a genetically different individual of the same species
Xenograft	Xenogeneic	Transplants between different species

Transplants can be broadly divided based on the genetic relationship between donor and recipient (Table 6-21).

The major indications for transplantation are listed in Table 6-22.

Transplantation immunology encompasses most aspects of the human immune response to antigens expressed by the donor organ or tissue. When donor and recipient genetic disparities exist, the recipient mounts a specific immune response to the antigens expressed by the donor grafted organ.

Despite the treatment of recipients with immunosuppressive drugs, the possibility of immunologic rejection exists. The types of rejection, their temporal relationship to the transplant, and their presumed pathologic mechanism are noted in Table 6-23.

Complications with transplantation are still frequent and require management. General complications can be broadly characterized into those caused by rejection (as above), medication-induced side effects, and complications induced by immunosuppression. Additionally, there are some organ-specific complications observed in certain types of transplantations. Many of the immunosuppressive medications are hepatotoxic and nephrotoxic.

TABLE 6–23: Rejection Of Transplants	
Type of Rejection	**Description**
Acute	Usually occurs within days to weeks owing to primary activation of the T-cell response
Chronic	Usually occurs months to years after transplantation; probably occurs by continued, albeit muted, cell-mediated toxicity and other unclear causes
Hyperacute	Usually occurs minutes to hours after transplantation and is caused by preformed antidonor antibodies activating complement

TABLE 6–22: Major Indications For Transplantation*			
Type of transplant	**Indication**	**Type of transplant**	**Indication**
Kidney	End-stage renal disease Glomerulonephritis Pyelonephritis Congenital abnormalities Nephrotic syndrome Renal tumor (eg. Wilms tumor in children or renal cell carcinoma in adults)	Liver	End-stage liver disease Primary biliary cirrhosis Biliary atresia (children) Chronic hepatitis Sclerosing cholangitis
Heart	Cardiomyopathy Severe coronary artery disease Congestive heart failure	Heart and lung	Multiorgan end-stage disease Congenital abnormalities Amyloidosis
Pancreas	Severe diabetes leading to renal disease	Lung	Primary pulmonary hypertension COPD/emphysema Pulmonary fibrosis Cystic fibrosis
Intestinal Non solid organ	Massive short bowel syndrome		
HSCT – hematopoietic stem cell transplantation (autologous)	Acute myelogenous leukemia, multiple myeloma and amyloidosis, lymphoma (Hodgkin and non-Hodgkin), possibly solid tumors (breast, germ cell, ovarian), SLE/autoimmune disorders	Hematopoietic stem cell transplantation (allogeneic)	Leukemia, lymphomas, multiple myeloma, aplastic anemia, primary immunodeficiencies, hemoglobinopathies (sickle cell, thalassemia),
COPD = chronic obstructive pulmonary disorder; SLE = systemic lupus erythematosus. *Partial listing only.			

TABLE 6–24: Outcomes of Solid Organ Transplantation					
	Type of Transplantation				
	Renal (Living Donor)	*Renal (Cadaveric)*	*Heart*	*Liver (Cadaveric)*	*Lung*
1 yr graft survival (%)	95	89	87	82	81
5 yr graft survival (%)	80	67	72	67	48
1 yr patient survival (%)	98	95	88	87	83
5 yr patient survival (%)	90	81	73	73	49
Data are from the 2005 annual report of the USSRTROPTN.2 (accessed July 2006).					

Many of the medications also alter the metabolism of drugs commonly used in dentistry. Immunosuppression renders the transplant patient susceptible to various infections, including bacterial, viral, and fungal infections. Opportunistic infections are also common. Immunosuppression also makes the transplant patient more susceptible to malignancies, including post-transplant lymphoproliferative disorders. A specific complication related to HSCT is graft-versus-host disease (GVHD), a condition in which allogeneic HCT recipients develop a complex immunologic phenomenon that occurs when immunocompetent cells from the donor are given to an immunodeficient host. The host, who possesses transplantation antigens foreign to the graft, stimulates an immune response by the newly en-grafted immune cells. GVHD affects the entire gastrointestinal system, including the mouth, as well as the skin and the liver. This reaction can be lethal and requires therapy with intensive immunosuppression. Chronic mucosal ulceration seen in GVHD may serve as an entry port for other infectious pathogens.

Although transplantation is fraught with complications related to rejection, it is still markedly successful. Outcomes of solid organ transplantation are listed in Table 6-24.

According to World Wide Network of Blood and Marrow Transplantation, more than 50,000 first HSCTs (53% autologous and 47% allogeneic) are performed every year worldwide. The annual rate of growth of this procedure has been estimated to between 10 and 20%. Improved HCT-related health care has resulted in less morbidity and lower mortality rates. Historically, HCTs for hematologic malignancies were undertaken as salvage therapy for refractory cancers, but outcomes are actually better for patients who are treated with HCT soon after diagnosis or in remission rather than after multiple relapses of hematologic disease. Outcomes have improved in both autologous and allogeneic HCTs.

Dental Management
Dental treatment for patients who are preparing for transplantation or for those who have had a transplant should be coordinated with the transplant physician. The treating dentist needs to remember that the patient may be a better candidate for elective dental treatment after the transplanted organ is stable. However, the patient's general dentist may be consulted before "listing" the patient for the Transplantation. The nature of this consultation is to ensure that the patient does not have any acute (or potentially acute) dental or oral infection that could complicate the transplantation process. It is prudent for a transplant candidate to be examined by the dentist in the pretransplantation period.

A dentist treating members of this unique population must be aware of certain considerations regarding the medical health of the individuals; providing dental care is often challenging. Dental management for this patient population can be divided into pretransplantation and post-transplantation issues, as noted in Table 6-25.

Oral lesions in this population include various infections, including opportunistic infections. Bacterial infections may be caused by bacteria not normally associated with oral infection. Viral infections include recurrent intraoral and labial herpetic simplex infections, cytomegalovirus infections, which clinically resemble deep aphthous-like ulcerations, and Epstein-Barr virus, which results in oral hairy leukoplakia. Epstein-Barr virus is also associated with post-transplant lymphoproliferative disorder. In addition to superficial fungal infections, such as candidiasis, deep fungal infections could also be present. On clinical examination, deep fungal infections tend to be necrotic plaques.

The dentist needs an exceptionally strong knowledge base in medicine to minimize adverse outcomes secondary to provision of oral health care for this unique population. It is essential that the dentist familiarize himself or herself with the special needs of these patients.

TABLE 6–25: Dental Management Considerations

Pre-Transplantation
 	
 • Significantly ill patient with end-organ damage
 • Medical consultation required
 • Consider postponing elective treatment
 • Dental consultation prior to anticipated transplantation
     Rule out dental infectious sources, definitively
     Perform necessary treatment; this will require consultation with a transplantation physician to determine medical risk-to-benefit ratio
     Obtain laboratory information/supplemental information as needed
     Become acquainted with specific management issues (e.g., blood products, prophylactic antibiotics) that may need to be employed if treatment is rendered

Post-Transplantation
 	
 • Immediate post-transplantation period
     No elective dental treatment performed
     Emergency treatment only with medical consultation and consideration of specific management needs
 • Stable post-transplantation period
     Elective treatment may be performed after medical consultation with the transplantation physician
     Issues of immunosuppression must be recognized
     Immunosuppressant medication interactions must be understood
     Oral mucosal disease and oral infections must be diagnosed and treated
     Supplemental corticosteroids (steroid boost) may be necessary
     Consideration of antibiotic prophylaxis needed
     Consideration of specific management needs based on the organ type of transplant
 • Post-transplantation chronic rejection period
     Only emergency treatment
     Patients are very ill as they are immunosuppressed and have organ failure

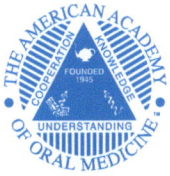

7 Neurologic Conditions

SEIZURE DISORDERS

Definition

A seizure is the result of spontaneous, uncontrollable, hypersynchronous discharge of cerebral neurons that may result in abrupt suspension of motor, sensory, behavioral, or body function. The term epilepsy is used to describe a chronic neurological condition characterized by recurrent unprovoked seizures. A convulsion is a physical sign of certain types of seizures characterized by excessive and abnormal muscle contractions.

Epidemiology

Globally, the annual incidence of epilepsy in high-income countries is between 30-50 per 100,000 people while in less developed countries, it can be up to 2 times higher.

In the United States, the annual incidence is estimated at approximately 48 per 100,000 people. The age-specific incidence has a bimodal distribution with higher rates found in children and the elderly compared with adults. It is estimated that 1 in 26 people will develop epilepsy over the course of their lifetime.

Classification of Seizures

TABLE 7-1: Classification of Seizures (Based on the 2010 ILAE Revised Classification System

1. Generalized seizures
  • Tonic-clonic
  • Absence
    • Typical
    • Atypical
  • Myoclonic
  • Atonic

2. Focal seizures
3. Unknown   • Epileptic spasms

The International League Against Epilepsy (ILAE) released a revised classification system for seizures and epilepsies in 2010. The revised classification system is presented in Table 7-1.

Seizures are subdivided into 3 categories: generalized, focal (formerly referred to as partial) and unknown, which includes epileptic spasms.

GENERALIZED SEIZURES

Generalized seizures originate within and rapidly engage bilateral distributed neuronal networks, which can be cortical or subcortical structures and do not necessarily need to involve the whole cortex. Generalized seizures are subdivided into tonic-clonic, absence, myoclonic and atonic seizures.

TONIC-CLONIC SEIZURES

Tonic-clonic seizures are characterized by a sudden loss of consciousness followed by muscular rigidity (tonic phase). Frequently, an aura precedes the onset of tonic-clonic seizures. Aura may consist of auditory, gustatory, and olfactory hallucinations; slurring of speech; frequent blinking; irritability; and/or mood changes. Following the tonic phase (generally lasting for < 1 minute), the clonic phase begins and is characterized by forceful jerking of the head, trunk, and extremities. This phase can last from a few seconds to several minutes. Once clonic activity has ceased, the patient enters the postictal phase, which is characterized by a slow return to consciousness, headache, disorientation, muscle soreness, and inclination toward sleep.

ABSENCE SEIZURES

Absence seizures are characterized by a very brief period (seconds) of unconsciousness without an absence of body tone. Patients can appear to be daydreaming, with an ability to resume motor and intellectual activity from the point these activities ceased owing to onset of seizure activity. Other features of absence seizures include rapid blinking of the eyelids, minor movements of the hands, and/or subtle facial twitching without generalized muscular activity.

Atypical absence seizures tend to begin more slowly and last longer than typical absence seizures. They are associated often with a loss of muscle tone and occur more commonly in individuals with intellectual impairment.

MYOCLONIC SEIZURES

A myoclonic seizure involves sudden, brief single or multiple muscle contractions without impairment of consciousness.

ATONIC SEIZURES

An atonic seizure involves loss of body tone without a preceding myoclonic or tonic episode.

FOCAL SEIZURES

Focal seizures, formally known as partial seizures originate in neuronal networks limited to one hemisphere. In the revised classification system, the terms simple partial, complex partial and secondarily generalized have been eliminated, as they were often misused and difficult to precisely define. Instead focal seizures are described based on their features. Examples of descriptors of focal seizures include:

- Without impairment of consciousness or awareness
- Involving subjective sensory or psychic phenomena only
- With impairment of consciousness or awareness
- Evolving to a bilateral convulsive seizure

UNKNOWN

This classification is used for seizure types where the underlying cause is unknown.

Pathogenesis

In the 2010 ILAE revised classification system, the use of the terms idiopathic, symptomatic and cryptogenic to describe the etiology of epilepsy was discontinued. Instead, the three classes of etiologies recommended are genetic, structural or metabolic and unknown. Genetic epilepsies are the result of a known or presumed genetic defect(s) in which the seizures are the primary symptom of the disorder. Structural and metabolic epilepsies involve distinct structural or metabolic abnormalities that are associated with an increased risk of epilepsy. Examples of structural or metabolic disorders that may result in epilepsy include trauma, infection, cerebral ischemia/hypoxia, hypoglycemia, convulsive drugs such as cocaine, and withdrawal from alcohol, barbiturates, and benzodiazepines. Other

causes include developmental anomalies, immune mediated disorders, metabolic defects, and diseases affecting the central nervous system (CNS), such as neoplasia and vascular malformations. The third class of etiology is unknown cause, which means that the nature of the underlying cause is not currently known.

Diagnosis

Diagnosis of seizure disorders includes a thorough medical evaluation, beginning with a complete medical history to determine the type, frequency, triggers, and events associated with the seizure activity. Medications should be reviewed as several types can induce seizure activity, including lidocaine and benzodiazepines. Physical examination findings may be helpful in determining underlying anomalies such as mental retardation. Laboratory tests should be used to rule out metabolic diseases that can induce seizure activity and include complete blood counts, electrolytes, calcium, magnesium, phosphorus, serum glucose values, and evaluation of cerebrospinal fluid, if indicated. Serum prolactin is usually elevated up to three fold immediately after an epileptic seizure and is useful in differentiating epileptic from non-epileptic/ psychogenic seizures. A complete neurologic examination should be completed, accompanied by diagnostic and imaging studies. The most valuable diagnostic study is an electroencephalogram, which is a recording of the electrical activity of the brain. It is useful for identifying seizure type and predicting the likelihood of recurrence. The imaging modality of choice is a magnetic resonance image, which can be supplemented by computed tomography to reveal structural abnormalities responsible for inducing seizure activity.

Medical Treatment

Elimination or control of underlying pathology is critical for treating recurrent seizure disorders with an identifiable etiology. Treatment of CNS infections, surgical removal of neoplasms, and correction of metabolic imbalances are frequently indicated. Patients may have an implanted vagus nerve stimulator to aid in preventing seizure activity. For patients with recurrent seizures without identifiable causative pathology or whose management is refractory to other means, pharmacologic therapy is initiated. The goal of pharmacologic therapy is to choose a drug that is most appropriate for the specific type of seizure activity and to administer it in the proper dose to achieve control of seizure activity with minimal side effects. (Table 7-2)

Physical Status

Approximately 60 to 70% of patients with idiopathic seizure disorders enter prolonged remission (> 5 years)

TABLE 7–2: Medications Often Used for Management of Seizure Disorders		
Medication	*Use*	*Possible Adverse Side Effects*
Levatiracetam (Keppra)	Myoclonic, focal and tonic-clonic seizures	Weakness, increased blood pressure, somnolence, infection, nasopharyngitis
Carbamazepine (Tegretol)	Primarily for focal seizures	Ataxia, dizziness, diplopia, agranulocytosis, thrombocytopenia, liver dysfunction
Clonazepam (Klonopin)	Primarily for absence seizures	General CNS depression, drowsiness, ataxia, abnormal behavior, palpitations, muscle weakness
Diazepam (Valium)	Status epilepticus	Drowsiness, fatigue, ataxia, headache, nausea
Ethosuximide (Zarontin)	Primarily for absence seizures	GI upset, somnolence, blood dyscrasias, gingival hypertrophy, tongue swelling
Lamotrigine (Lamictal)	Primarily for focal seizures	Dizziness, ataxia, somnolence, headache, diplopia, blurred vision, nausea, vomiting, rash
Midazolam (Versed)	Status epilepticus	Respiratory depression, decreased blood pressure, nausea, vomiting, diplopia, mood swings
Phenytoin (Dilantin)	Tonic-clonic seizures	Confusion, lethargy, ataxia, gingival hyperplasia/overgrowth, blood dyscrasias, skin rash, allergic reaction
Phenobarbital	Tonic-clonic seizures	Drowsiness, CNS depression, megaloblastic anemia (rare)
Topiramate (Topamax)	Tonic-clonic seizures	Mood disturbances, confusion, sedation, paresthesias, hyperthermia, acidosis
Valproic acid (Depakene) Divalproex sodium (Depakote)	Absence seizures, focal seizures with loss of consciousness	GI upset such as indigestion, nausea, vomiting, hypersalivation, anorexia, increased appetite, cramping, diarrhea, and constipation
CNS = central nervous system; GI = gastrointestinal.		

with use of antiseizure medications. Nearly 50% of these patients eventually become seizure free. Approximately 30% of patients continue to have seizures and never achieve remission, especially those with severe epilepsy that began in childhood. Patients with seizures secondary to acquired brain injuries or developmental abnormalities may have impaired cognitive function. Overall, patients with seizure disorders are at risk of developing psychiatric problems and short-term memory loss that may progress over time. Status epilepticus is a condition that refers to generalized tonic-clonic seizures that do not abate spontaneously (i.e., continuous seizure activity exceeding 5 minutes) or recur without the patient regaining consciousness. It is considered a medical emergency owing to the possible serious adverse sequelae of this condition, including aspiration, cardiac arrhythmias, bodily injury, and permanent neurologic damage.

Dental Management
A thorough evaluation of a patient's seizure disorder is necessary prior to initiation of any dental treatment. Important aspects to evaluate include the type of seizures, etiology of seizures, frequency of seizures, known triggers of seizure activity, presence of aura prior to seizure activity, compliance to medications and history of injuries related to seizure activity. Patients with a stable seizure disorder and no associated risks can receive outpatient dental care. If a patient demonstrates signs of poorly or uncontrolled seizure disorder, consultation with the patient's physician and/or neurologist is recommended to determine stability and the appropriate venue in which to receive dental care. Patients with poorly or uncontrolled seizure disorder may be referred to a hospital setting for routine dental care.

Dental care should include avoidance of any known triggers of the patient's seizure activity. Patients with poorly controlled seizures or with stress-triggered seizures may require sedative medications prior to treatment. Minimize the risk of injury and aspiration during dental treatment via dental floss–secured mouth props (which are easily

TABLE 7–3: Special Considerations for Seizure Disorders	
Concern	*Management*
Patients taking CNS depressants	Avoid or reduce dosage of narcotics
Patients with a history of lidocaine sensitivity	Avoid use in susceptible patients
Patients with foreign bodies in the mouth	Remove all loose objects from the mouth
Uncontrollable seizure activity	Gently restrain the patient, position the patient on the side, and lift the jaw to avoid aspiration; monitor vital signs
CNS = central nervous system.	

TABLE 7–4: Status Epilepticus
Treatment of status epilepticus (continuous seizure activity exceeding 5 min):
• Activate emergency medical services
• Administer intranasal midazolam 2 to 5 mg, lorazepam 4 to 8 mg (0.05 to 0.1 mg/kg) or diazepam 10 mg
• Alternatively, slow IV injection of midazolam 2 to 5 mg (or more), lorazepam 4 to 8 mg (0.05 to 0.1 mg/kg) or diazepam 10 mg until seizure activity stops
• If IV access is not possible, intramuscular diazepam / midazolam may be required

retrievable) and use of a rubber dam. If a patient experiences a seizure while receiving dental treatment, it is critical to remove all objects from the patient's mouth and to protect the patient from the surrounding environment. Vital signs should be assessed, airway support should be provided (if necessary), and the patient should be monitored to ensure that seizure activity ceases within a reasonable period of time. Tonic-clonic seizures usually last 1-3 minutes. (Tables 7-3 and 7-4).

Anti-seizure medications can significantly impact oral tissues and induce blood dyscrasias. Patients taking phenytoin may exhibit some degree of gingival overgrowth, and surgical debridement or excision may be indicated for removal of the excess tissue. In addition, antiseizure medications may cause hyposalivation, which can increase susceptibility to dental caries and candidiasis. Patients at high risk for development of dental caries may benefit from frequent recall visits and periodic applications of topical fluoride. Patients should be monitored regularly for signs and symptoms of candidiasis and should be treated with antifungals when indicated. Patients taking phenytoin, carbamazepine, valproic acid and ethosuximide may develop leukopenia and thrombocytopenia; these patients may be at increased risk of microbial infection, delayed healing, and bleeding complications. A complete blood count with differential is indicated prior to dental treatment to assess white blood cell and platelet counts. Patients with severe neutropenia (neutrophils < 500 per cc)

should have elective dental treatment postponed until their counts return to normal. Antibiotic prophylaxis and perioperative antibiotics should be considered if dental care must be provided to a patient who has significant neutropenia. Patients with significant thrombocytopenia (< 50,000 platelets per cc) generally require infusion of platelets prior to surgical procedures. Valproic acid inhibits the secondary phase of platelet aggregation and can result in prolonged bleeding; coagulation studies are recommended prior to surgical procedures. Local measures (sutures, cellulose matrix) should be considered to aid in hemostasis. Aspirin and nonsteroidal anti-inflammatory medications should be avoided for postoperative pain control in patients taking valproic acid as this interaction can increase the possibility of increased bleeding.

MULTIPLE SCLEROSIS
Definition
Multiple sclerosis (MS) is a chronic, autoimmune, inflammatory demyelinating disease characterized by the presence of progressive neurologic symptoms involving the CNS, optic nerve, and spinal cord. An estimated 2.3 million people live with MS worldwide and it typically presents in adults between 20 and 50 years of age with women affected twice as much as men. The cause is unknown but it has been linked to infectious, environmental and genetic factors. Areas of demyelination or plaques occur in the white matter of the CNS with a strong presence of inflammatory mediators, cytokines, and lymphocytes, which contribute

to the destruction of myelin. The clinical course of the disease is classified into four major categories:

- Clinically Isolated Syndrome (CIS): describes the first clinical presentation of neurologic signs and symptoms characteristic of inflammatory demyelination, which does not yet meet the criteria for diagnosis as MS

- Relapsing-Remitting MS (RRMS): the most common form characterized by periods of relapses marked by exacerbation of symptoms followed by periods of remission without disease progression

- Secondary Progressive MS (SPMS): a progression of RRMS with steady worsening of symptoms with or without periods of remission

- Primary Progressive MS (PPMS): in which symptoms continue to gradually worsen and decline from onset of MS

Physical Evaluation

MS patients present with various neurological symptoms including fatigue, spasticity mostly affecting the legs, sensory disturbances leading to loss of limb perception, gait and balance alterations, vision problems (optic neuritis, diplopia, nystagmus), dizziness, vertigo, dysphagia, slurred speech, bowel and bladder incontinence, chronic pain, facial pain with features similar to trigeminal neuralgia and emotional disturbances including depression.

Diagnosis is reached by exclusion and includes careful consideration of the history, presenting signs and symptoms, findings on imaging studies (magnetic resonance imaging), cerebrospinal fluid (CSF) analysis and sensory evoked potential tests. The CSF in multiple sclerosis patients is positive for bands of immunoglobulins known as oligoclonal bands. Suspicion of other pathology is high if any of the following are found during history and physical examination: symptoms can be explained by localized disease, absence of remission periods, normal laboratory findings, and sparing of optic, sensory, or bladder innervations.

Medical Treatment

Treatment is directed to the underlying immune disorder as well as associated symptoms and complications. Elevated doses of corticosteroids are given to control acute exacerbations and reduce neural inflammation. Immunomodulating therapy has become more common owing to the associated side effects of the chronic use of corti-

costeroids. Currently, corticosteroids are limited only to acute exacerbations. Interferon-β and glatiramer acetate have replaced corticosteroids in chronic dosing. Although current evidence suggests the high efficacy of these medications, they also carry serious side effects. Treatment with interferon can cause flu-like symptoms, malaise, myalgia, fever, and joint pains, whereas glatiramer acetate can cause blushing, shortness of breath, and palpitations. Other medications used in the treatment of this condition include biologic agents (natalizumab, alemtuzumab and daclizumab), as well as the antineoplastic agent mitoxantrone, which has been reported to increase risk for leukemia and induce cardiotoxic effects.

Physical Status: Severity

Multiple sclerosis varies in severity and speed of progression. Recuperation periods between attacks become shorter as the disease runs its course, and limb weakness tends to remain in the late stages. As an average, the disease can have a clinical course of up to 35 years, with milestones at years 15 and 25, when neurologic symptoms worsen. Assessment of the severity of the condition must be done based on the frequency, number, and characteristics of the attacks and length of time since diagnosis.

Dental Management

BEFORE TREATMENT: The dental professional should be aware of the clinical course of the disease and perform a risk assessment at the time of consultation, in cooperation with the treating neurologist. Patients with severe disease who cannot tolerate treatment in an out-patient setting may be referred to a hospital setting for dental treatment under sedation. The patient's motor and perceptual ability, especially in the facial area, must be evaluated prior to initiating invasive surgical procedures. Of note is the reported appearance of bilateral trigeminal neuralgia symptoms in multiple sclerosis patients. Patients below the age of 30 years who present with trigeminal neuralgia should receive an evaluation for multiple sclerosis. In light of the severe side effects of acute corticosteroid dosing, the clinician should consult the treating physician owing to the risk of adrenal suppression.

DURING TREATMENT: The side effects of medications used for treatment of multiple sclerosis as well as possible interactions with medications routinely used in the dental practice must be kept in mind.

AFTER TREATMENT: Patients with gait alterations or leg weakness should be monitored or helped while walking to prevent a fall. (See Table 7-5)

TABLE 7–5: Pharmacologic Therapy for Multiple Sclerosis Patients: Dental Considerations
Be aware of potential side effects, especially the presence of cardiovascular manifestations
Routine complete blood count is suggested for patients on frequent interferon therapy; monitor white blood cell count for immunosuppression
Monitor for signs or symptoms of chronic corticosteroid therapy, including unstable blood pressure, peptic ulcer disease, behavioral alterations, osteoporosis, and adrenal suppression

ALZHEIMER DISEASE

Definition

Alzheimer disease (AD) is a common form of dementia (responsible for almost half of dementia cases) characterized by progressive cognitive, functional and behavioral impairment. An estimated 5.4 million Americans and 48 million people worldwide have AD and these numbers continue to increase rapidly due to the aging of the population. One in 9 individuals over the age of 65 years and one in 3 individuals over the age of 85 years will present with clinical signs and symptoms consistent with the disease. Sporadic AD, also known as late-onset AD accounts for the majority of cases and usually manifests after age 65. Familial AD is a rare form of the disease with early-onset before age 65 and an autosomal dominant inheritance pattern. Presumed risk factors include reduced brain reserve capacity, decreased mental and physical activity in late life, low mental ability in early life, high cholesterol, hypertension, atherosclerosis, and previous head trauma. AD is characterized by the appearance of neuritic plaques and tangles in the medial temporal lobe structures and cortical brain areas. The etiology of the disease has been postulated as associated with amyloid production and metabolism in the brain.

Physical Evaluation

Clinical presentation includes loss of episodic memory, aphasia, impaired judgment and decision making, and disorientation. Initial changes affect the ability to judge time, and remembering names, words and tasks. At the advanced stages of the disease patients may experience extreme mood swings, confusion, hallucinations, weight loss and incontinence. There is a significant association between the amount of plaque and tangles and the severity of the disease in younger patients. The diagnosis of AD is made primarily by exclusion and is reached by combination of the history, clinical findings, and neurological examination. Investigations to rule out other causes of dementia include complete blood count, metabolic panel, serum B12 and folate levels, thyroid function tests, urinalysis, infection screening and neuroimaging studies such as CT and MRI. Additional diagnostic studies include amyloid β positron emission tomography, CSF analysis, electroencephalography (EEG) and genotyping for apoliprotein E. Diagnostic confirmation is possible only with brain biopsy or at autopsy.

Medical Treatment

Acetylcholinesterase inhibitors are used in an attempt to reduce symptoms. Memantine, an N-methyl-D-aspartate receptor antagonist is used for the management of moderate to severe AD. Psychotropic medications such as antidepressants and anxiolytics are used to treat the secondary symptoms of the disease. Other medications include antioxidants such as Vitamin E and seleginine, anti-inflammatory agents, estrogen and herbal remedies such as Ginkgo biloba. (See Table 7-6)

TABLE 7–6: Pharmacologic Management of Alzheimer Disease	
Drug	**Interaction**
Donezepil	CYP2D6/CYP3A4 interaction
Galantamine	CYP2D6/CYP3A4 interaction
Rivastigmine	No CYP interaction
Memantine	No CYP interaction

Physical Status: Severity

The severity and progression of the disease are assessed by psychiatric standardized testing (cognitive and functional) and progressive increments of symptoms.

Dental Management

BEFORE TREATMENT: The clinician should assess the cognitive levels and ability to consent to and withstand dental treatment. Patients with severe memory and behavioral issues are not candidates for outpatient dental care.

DURING TREATMENT: Patients should be treated with empathy and respect. The dentist should engage the patient's attention, listen carefully and reassure the patient constantly.

All procedure should be carefully explained using short sentences. Caution must be taken with rotary instrumentation. Some patients may require light or conscious sedation to provide safe care. The facial appearance of AD patients may be clinically similar to that of myasthenia or dystonia patients.

AFTER TREATMENT: Caution should be taken with medications that are prescribed to patients taking Donezepil or Galantamine, which are metabolized by CYP enzymes.

PARKINSON DISEASE (PD)
Definition
Parkinson disease is a progressive neurodegenerative disorder resulting from reduced dopaminergic neurons in the substantia nigra of the brain. It is characterized by motor, sensory, and cognitive impairment. Resting tremor, and bradykinesia are pathognomonic of the condition (Table 7-7).

TABLE 7–7: Features of Parkinson Disease
Bradykinesia
Resting tremor
Postural instability
Rigidity

PD is the second most common neurodegenerative disorder after Alzheimer disease. Approximately 10 million people globally and 1 million Americans live with PD. The prevalence of the disease is less than 1% of the population below the age of 50 years, 1% of the population older than 60 years and up to 4% of the population older than 80 years. There is no clear gender predilection, although current evidence of male preponderance is weak. Pathologic changes include neuronal loss and changes in the substantia nigra of the brain. These changes correspond to the onset of loss of motor coordination and subsequent behavioral and cognitive alterations, secondary to a deficiency of the potent neurotransmitter dopamine. Although a specific etiology has not been described, environmental effects and genetic susceptibility are believed to trigger the disease. Exposure to pesticides and brain trauma also are contributory.

Physical Evaluation
Physical evaluation of the patient who has PD requires assessment of motor skills in the early stages of the disease and cognitive or behavioral assessment during disease progression. Brain imaging is used as a supplemental tool to assess progression and prognosis. The diagnosis of PD is mostly based on the onset of clinical characteristics and the response to levodopa. Definitive diagnosis, in many cases, can be confirmed only by long-term patient follow-up.

Medical Treatment
Medical management of PD is based on disease staging. A pharmacologic approach is widely used, and there is some evidence on the efficacy of surgical interventions (Table 7-8).

TABLE 7–8: Medical Management of Parkinson Disease	
Drugs	**Stages**
Monoamine oxidase Type B Inhibitor (e.g., selegiline)	
Anticholinergics (e.g., amantadine)	Early stage
Serotonin reuptake inhibitors	
Dopamine agonists (mono- or combined therapy)	Intermediate stage
Levodopa/carbidopa	Late stage
Catecol O-methyltransferase (COMT) inhibitors	

Physical Status: Severity
Similar to other neurodegenerative disorders, physical status and the severity of the condition are determined by symptomatic function and cognitive testing.

Dental Management
BEFORE TREATMENT: A thorough medical history is required to assess disease status and control. Patients in advanced stages of the disease may require moderate physical restrictions or sedation to limit involuntary movements and tremors. The hallmark of care is prevention and caregiver recruitment into the oral care routine if the patient is unable to adequately perform self–oral care.

DURING TREATMENT: Patient positioning in the dental chair is important. In addition to chorea, some patients may express tardive dyskinesia (involuntary muscle movement secondary to PD or anti-psychotic drug therapies) of the facial and neck muscles. Owing to rigidity, patients may need to be seen in a wheelchair. Medication interactions are important to remember (e.g., COMT inhibitors and epinephrine in a local anesthetic; recommend limiting to two carpules of 1:100,000 epinephrine), as well as possible CNS depression caused by certain medications used for PD. Long-term treatment with levodopa can exacerbate tremors, dyskinesia, and imbalance owing to increased tolerance.

AFTER TREATMENT: Patients may suffer from xerostomia or severe sialorrhea owing to swallowing impairment and rigidity. Salivary replacement therapy can be used for xerostomic patients, as well as home fluoride therapy.

MYASTHENIA GRAVIS

Definition

Myasthenia gravis is an autoimmune disorder characterized by the presence of antibodies against acetylcholine receptors. Consequently, there is an autoimmune destruction of multiple neuronal synapses. The prevalence of the disorder in the United States is estimated at 14 to 20 per 100 000 population, with a marked female preference. The mean age at onset is around 30 years in women and 60 years in men. Almost any muscular group can be affected.

Physical Evaluation

Symptoms include extreme muscle weakness. Eighty to 90% of patients present with circulating antibodies against acetylcholine receptors. Symptom intensity changes during the day and depends on the extent of involvement. Muscles of the face present tone changes (drooping, dropped jaw) and a mask-like expression. Ocular involvement leads to diplopia. Ocular symptoms occur as an initial presentation in 50% of patients but occur in 90% of patients during the course of the illness. The critical and most serious period of clinical complications is in the initial 3 years after diagnosis. It is worth noting that a small percentage (15%) of patients may develop either thymic hyperplasia or thymoma. A similar percentage has been linked to the appearance of other autoimmune disease involving endocrine organs or hematopoiesis. The diagnosis of myasthenia gravis is reached by a detailed physical examination, electromyography, and specialized tests that measure cholinesterase activity. Serologic testing measures antibody binding to tagged acetylcholinesterase receptors. This test is sensitive to moderate and severe disease and less effective in patients suffering from mild disease or only limited muscular involvement. However, a small number of patients can have negative serology. Chest CT or MRI is important to rule out thymic disease.

Medical Treatment

The first line of therapy is given by cholinesterase inhibitors such as pyridostigmine. This approach is particularly effective early in the disease. Although remission can be observed short term, continuous treatment with this medication requires escalating doses. Once the maximum dose is given, most patients will become refractory to its effects. Ephedrine, 3,4-diaminopyridine, and medications (penicillamine and aminoglycosides) have an effect at the neuromuscular junction. Elevated doses of corticosteroids are commonly given to these patients to achieve remission. Azathioprine has been used as a single agent or in combination with low-dose corticosteroids. Plasmapheresis, intravenous immunoglobulin newer monoclonal antibodies such as rituximab and thymectomy have proven effective.

Physical Status: Severity

The physical status of the myasthenia gravis patient is assessed from the muscle groups involved, length of time since diagnosis, and symptoms. The morbidity and mortality of this condition have decreased greatly with advances in management of the disorder. However, as a chronic autoimmune condition, compromised respiratory muscles and/or neck muscles are the hallmarks for late stages of the disease.

Dental Management

BEFORE TREATMENT: Dental care of these patients should be provided close to the time of medication intake (close to the half-life of the medication) to take advantage of symptom control. A detailed medication list should be provided, as well as timing. Patients taking corticosteroids or immunosuppressants should provide a recent complete blood count to assess leukopenia. The potential for adrenal suppression must be evaluated, considering the time and amount of medication. Supplemental corticosteroids may be needed for extensive oral surgical procedures.

DURING TREATMENT: Careful attention must be paid to respiratory drive. To avoid aspiration, use of rubber dam and efficient suctioning is recommended. Patients at advanced stages should have pulse oximeter monitoring and be seen in a hospital setting. Muscarinic side effects may be seen intraorally (excessive saliva) secondary to cholinesterase inhibitors.

AFTER TREATMENT: Caution must be taken with prescribing of narcotic medications. Patients on corticosteroids should be given nonsteroidal anti-inflammatory drugs with caution owing to gastric irritation. Alternative pain control medications are recommended.

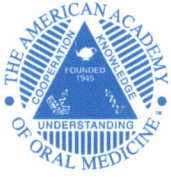

8 Pregnancy and Breast Feeding

Although not a medical complication per se, pregnancy imposes specific physiologic stressors on the gravid patient. Clinicians have an obligation to provide safe and effective dental care that addresses the mother's oral heath care needs while also ensuring the safety of the developing fetus. In addition to considering the mother's ability to tolerate the stress associated with a given dental procedure, the clinician must consider its impact on the developing fetus. This is especially true with regard to medications, which may be distributed from the maternal plasma through the placenta to the fetus or to breast milk, which may be ingested by the newborn infant during nursing.

Physiology

Following fertilization, a hormonally directed cascade of physiologic changes ensues, all focused on the nurturing and ultimate delivery of new life. The production of maternal hormones increases, and placental hormone synthesis begins. Large amounts of estrogen and progesterone are secreted, along with growth hormone, insulin, vitamin D, cortisol, aldosterone, and thyroid hormones.

The physiologic changes associated with pregnancy affect virtually all body systems, including the cardiovascular, hematopoietic, respiratory, renal, and gastrointestinal systems. Increased water retention results in a 1 to 2 L expansion (30–50%) of blood volume. Cardiac output is increased 30 to 50%. Red blood cell production is increased (20–30%) but fails to keep pace with the blood volume expansion, resulting in a lowered hematocrit (dilutional anemia). Tachycardia, heart murmur, increased venous pressure, and potential vasomotor instability may occur. Reduced respiratory capacity leads to dyspnea and hyperventilation. Renal changes include a 30 to 50% increase in the glomerular filtration rate, increased urinary frequency, increased urgency, increased incontinence, and increased infection risk. Nausea, vomiting, and other dyspeptic symptoms (increased salivation, heartburn) are common in pregnancy and affect between 50 and 90% of women.

Increased appetite and cravings for unusual combinations of foods are common and may lead to dietary changes that are not nutritionally sound.

Physical Evaluation

Typically, the first clue to pregnancy is a missed menstrual cycle. Confirmatory laboratory tests all measure the level of human chorionic gonadotropin, a hormone that is produced by the placenta when a woman is pregnant. Most tests are ordered 10 days after the first missed period. Other signs and symptoms of pregnancy include fatigue, swollen or tender breasts, nausea or morning sickness, backache, headache, and dietary cravings. Once pregnancy is confirmed, the patient typically undergoes a thorough medical history review and physical evaluation to identify any comorbidities or potential complicating factors.

Medical Management and Complications

During pregnancy, the physical well-being of the patient is monitored closely with particular attention to her weight, blood pressure, and blood and urine profiles. Complications are infrequent when a healthy mother is afforded proper prenatal care. However, the two most commonly observed complications are preeclampsia and gestational diabetes mellitus (GDM).

Preeclampsia is a rapidly progressive condition characterized by hypertension and proteinuria. Hypertension is considered severe if there is sustained systolic elevation > 160 mm Hg and/or sustained diastolic elevation > 110 mm Hg. Hypertension associated with preeclampsia and eclampsia typically occurs after the twentieth week of gestation. Maternal complications include abruptio placentae, disseminated coagulopathy, pulmonary edema, acute renal failure, hepatic failure, stroke, long-term cardiovascular morbidity, eclampsia, and death. Fetal complications include preterm delivery, fetal growth restriction, hypoxic neurologic injury, long-term cardiovascular morbidity associated with low birth weight, and perinatal death. Proper medical management is predicated on a timely diagnosis.

GDM occurs in up to 7% of pregnancies and is defined as any degree of glucose intolerance with onset or first recognition during pregnancy. A fasting plasma glucose level > 126 mg/dL or a casual plasma glucose > 200 mg/dL meets the threshold for the diagnosis. Risk factors for GDM include marked obesity, high thyroid levels, an antecedent history of GDM and/or glycosuria, and a strong family history of diabetes mellitus. The presence of fasting hyperglycemia (> 105 mg/dL) may be associated with an increased risk of intrauterine fetal death during the last 4 to 8 weeks of gestation.

Common head and neck complications associated with pregnancy include pregnancy gingivitis, pregnancy tumor, tooth mobility, dental caries, and melasma. Pregnancy gingivitis and/or pregnancy tumors are associated with increased levels of proinflammatory mediators, which may increase the risk of preterm delivery and low birth weight. Tooth mobility may also be associated with inflammatory gingival changes but typically resolves following parturition. Dental caries during pregnancy is likely attributable to inadequate oral hygiene in conjunction with dietary cravings for carbohydrate-containing foods. Cariogenic bacteria, such as *Actinomyces naeslundii*, may initiate the release of proinflammatory mediators, which may increase the risk of preterm delivery and low birth weight. Melasma (chloasma) occurs in up to 75% of pregnant women and is characterized by hyperpigmentation of sun-exposed areas of the face, neck, and forearms. Melasma may persist postpartum.

Dental Management
The goals are to provide timely preventive and therapeutic strategies to the pregnant or nursing mother that are consistent with the patient's physical and emotional ability to undergo and respond to dental treatment, the patient's psychosocial needs, and the safety and well-being of the developing fetus or newborn. A consultation with the patient's physician is warranted to determine the patient's risk status prior to the initiation of required dental treatment, to relay relevant information to the physician about the dental needs of the patient and any proposed therapeutic interventions, and to reinforce the clinician's concern for the mother and her developing child. It is essential to monitor the patient's blood pressure, pulse, and respirations at each appointment. To maximize patient comfort, appointments should be shortened or the patient afforded frequent breaks. The pregnant patient is at risk for supine hypotensive syndrome, a condition in which

the gravid uterus impinges on the inferior vena cava and interrupts return blood flow to the heart. It is prevented by close intraoperative monitoring and having the patient use a pillow to elevate her right hip and/or slightly roll to the left while in the dental chair, thereby reducing uterine pressure on the inferior vena cava.

A preventive program consisting of oral hygiene instruction, dietary counseling, prophylaxis, and localized scaling as needed should be instituted during the first trimester of pregnancy and continued until after parturition. Practicing diligent oral hygiene reduces the risk of pregnancy gingivitis, pregnancy tumor, tooth mobility, and dental caries. Emergency dental care should be provided as needed to remediate pain and infection, but elective care is best deferred until after parturition. The pregnant patient is often acutely concerned about the risks associated with dental radiography. The estimated radiation exposure to the fetus associated with a full-mouth series and panoramic radiograph are 10–5 Gy and 15 x 10–5 Gy, respectively. In contrast, the estimated daily radiation background exposure is 4 x 10–4 Gy. Although the patient may be reassured that fetal exposure from dental radiographs is far lower than that from naturally occurring background radiation, informed consent should be obtained, and it is prudent to avoid or minimize the use of diagnostic radiography during pregnancy. This is especially true for the first trimester, when organogenesis occurs.

Ideally, drug administration can be avoided during pregnancy and nursing. If pharmacologic intervention becomes necessary, the clinician should obtain informed consent and only prescribe drugs that have the best documented pregnancy-associated profile (Table 8 -1) provides the Food and Drug Administration (FDA) safety criteria regarding drugs commonly used in dentistry.

In 2015, the Food and Drug Administration (FDA) proposed a change to this pregnancy labeling of drugs. The FDA Pregnancy and Lactation Labeling Rule (PLLR) proposes to replace the current letter category (A, B, C, D and X) with more relevant and critical information to aid in decision-making when prescribing drugs to pregnant or lactating women. The goal is to remove the pregnancy letter category by 2020. At this time, clinicians should be aware of both grading systems until the letter category is eliminated. Readers are encouraged to visit the FDA website (www.FDA.gov) and search for "PLLR" for detailed information, and to consult with the patient's obstetrician/gynecologist (OB/GYN) when prescribing medications to pregnant and lactating women, when needed.

CATEGORY A: Adequate, well-controlled studies in pregnant women have not shown an increased risk of fetal abnormalities.

CATEGORY B: Animal studies have revealed no evidence of harm to the fetus; however, there are no adequate and well-controlled studies in pregnant women.

    OR

Animal studies have shown an adverse effect, but adequate and well-controlled studies in pregnant women have failed to demonstrate a risk to the fetus.

CATEGORY C: Animal studies have shown an adverse effect, and there are no adequate and well-controlled studies in pregnant women.

    OR

No animal studies have been conducted, and there are no adequate and well-controlled studies in pregnant women.

CATEGORY D: Studies, adequate, well controlled, or observational, in pregnant women have demonstrated a risk to the fetus. However, the benefit of therapy may outweigh the potential risk.

CATEGORY X: Studies, adequate, well controlled, or observational, in animals or pregnant women have demonstrated positive evidence of fetal abnormalities. The use of the product is contraindicated in women who are or may become pregnant.

TABLE 8–1: Considerations in Drug Use During Pregnancy		
Therapeutic Agents	*FDA Category*	*During Lactation*
Anxiolytic agents		
Diphenhydramine	C	Use with caution
Benzodiazepines	D	Avoid
Barbiturates	D	Avoid
Nitrous oxide	Avoid using beyond 30 minutes	Safe
Local anesthetic agents*		
Lidocaine	B	Safe
Mepivacaine	C	Safe
Benzocaine	C	Safe
Analgesics		
APAP	B	Safe
Ibuprofen	B (D 3rd trimester)	Safe
Oxycodone	B	Avoid
ASA	C (D 3rd trimester)	Avoid
Codeine	C (D 3rd trimester)	Use with caution
Tramadol	C	Use with caution
Antimicrobials		
Pencillins	B	Safe
Cephalosporins	B	Safe
Clindamycin	B	Safe
Metronidazole	B	Safe
APAP = N-acetyl-p-aminophenol; ASA = acetylsalicylic acid; FDA = Food and Drug Administration. *The use of local anesthetic agents with epinephrine (< 0.1 mg bolus dose) is considered safe in a healthy pregnant patient.		

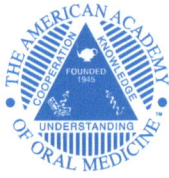

9 Dental Management of the Cancer Patient

Cancer has a profound individual and societal impact, with approximately 1,300,000 new cases diagnosed each year and an overall 5-year survival rate of 60%. Cancer is the second leading cause of death, accounting for approximately 1 in 7 deaths in the United States and a staggering overall cost of $180 billion.

With more than 1 million new cases of cancer diagnosed each year and a shift to outpatient management, it is likely that all dentists will see cancer patients under active care in their practice. Medically necessary oral care before, during, and after cancer treatment can prevent or reduce the incidence and severity of oral complications, enhancing both patient survival and quality of life. An active role by dentists in the management of patients with cancer produces benefits well beyond the oral cavity. Table 9-1 presents current information on the annual incidence of new cases of the most common cancers.

Each year, approximately 9,700 people die from oral cancer, and of the 49,500 individuals who are newly diagnosed with oral cancer, roughly half will be alive in 5 years. These numbers have not significantly improved in decades. The death rate associated with oral cancer is particularly high owing to the cancer being routinely discovered late in its development. Often oral cancer is discovered only after it has metastasized to another location. Early detection of oral cancer is one of the most beneficial diagnostic services that dentists can provide.

Often oral cancer develops because of lifestyle factors such as tobacco use and excessive alcohol consumption. Consequently, many cancers can be prevented through behavioral changes, such as reduction or elimination of tobacco use, which dentists can help promote.

BASICS OF CANCER MANAGEMENT

One of the first priorities in patient management after the diagnosis of cancer is established is to determine the extent of

TABLE 8–1: Estimated New Cancer Cases and Death in 2018 by Sex*					
Males	*New Cases*	*Deaths*	*Female*	*New Cases*	*Deaths*
Prostate	164,690	29,430	Breast	266,120	40,920
Lung & bronchus	121,680	83,550	Lung & bronchus	112,350	70,500
Urinary bladder	62,380	12,520	Uterine corpus	63,230	11,350
Melanoma of the skin	55,150	5,990	Thyroid	40,900	1,100
Kidney & renal pelvis	42,680	10,010	Melanoma of the skin	36,120	3,330
Non-Hodgkin lymphoma	41,730	11,510	Non-Hodgkin lymphoma	32,950	8,400
Oral cavity & pharynx	37,160	7280	Leukemia	25,270	10,100
Leukemia	35,030	14,270	Kidney & renal pelvis	22,660	4,960
Pancreas	29,200	23,020	Ovary	22,240	14,070
Colon & rectum	2960	480	Colon & rectum	5,620	680
* Siegel A et al. Cancer Statistics, 2018. CA Cancer J Clin 68:7-30, 2018.					

the disease. This process is called staging, and it is accomplished by a variety of noninvasive and invasive diagnostic tests and procedures. The most widely used system of staging is the TNM (tumor, node, metastasis) classification developed by the International Union Against Cancer and the American Joint Committee on Cancer.

Cancer treatments are divided into four main groups: surgery, radiation therapy (including photodynamic therapy), chemotherapy (including hormonal therapy), and biologic therapy (including immunotherapy, bone marrow transplantation, and agents targeting cancer cell biology). These modalities are often used in combination. The type of therapy for the malignancy depends on the specific diagnosis, site, and staging. Surgery and radiation therapy are considered local treatments, whereas chemotherapy and biologic therapy are usually systemic treatments.

From a dental management perspective, each type of cancer and each form of therapy requires a somewhat modified approach. It should be evident that the topic of dental management of the cancer patient is very broad. Because of this complexity, the subjects of oral cancer and cancer in general are covered in depth in separate monographs in the American Academy of Oral Medicine's Clinician Guides series. This chapter focuses on only two basic aspects of this important problem:

- Dental evaluation and treatment of patients with cancer prior to cancer therapy

- Dental treatment of patients after cancer therapy

DENTAL EVALUATION AND TREATMENT OF PATIENTS WITH CANCER PRIOR TO CANCER THERAPY
Importance of Pretreatment Dental Care
A thorough oral evaluation by a knowledgeable dental professional before cancer treatment begins is important to the success of therapy. Oral problems such as infection, nonrestorable teeth, fractured teeth or restorations, or periodontal disease that can contribute to oral complications during and after cancer therapy should be identified and treated. To ensure the best possible care, the dental team should work with the oncologist to learn the patient's cancer diagnosis, medical history, and treatment plan. Such open communication between providers improves the likelihood that the patient will successfully complete his or her cancer regimen.

Pre-Cancer Treatment Oral Health Examination
The pretreatment evaluation should include a thorough examination of hard and soft tissues, as well as appropriate radiographs, to detect possible sources of infection that could complicate or delay cancer therapy or create post treatment problems.

It is essential to identify and eliminate potential sites of infection, severely broken down teeth, periodontally compromised teeth, and tissue injury or trauma, including orthodontic bands and brackets, if highly stomatotoxic chemotherapy is planned or if the appliances will be in the radiation field.

A prosthodontic evaluation is indicated when prostheses are worn. The prosthesis should be well adapted to the tissue and removed from the mouth at night. Patients receiving radiation therapy or highly stomatotoxic chemotherapy will not be able to wear their prosthesis while under active care.

Table 9-2 lists some of the important pretreatment considerations when evaluating a patient who is to receive chemotherapy or radiation therapy.

TABLE 9-2: SPECIFIC PRETREATMENT CONSIDERATIONS	
When Chemotherapy Is Planned*	*Head and Neck Radiation Therapy* †
Consult with oncologist	Consult with radiation oncologist
Determine hematologic status	Determine extent of targeted tissue
Assess potential for bleeding problems	Find total dose of radiation therapy
Check for presence of central venous catheter	Inquire about other planned treatment
Determine schedule of care	Ask start date of radiation therapy

* Oral complications of chemotherapy depend on the specific cancer being treated, drugs used, dosages, degree of dental disease, and potential adjuvant radiation therapy.

† Patients receiving radiation therapy to the head and neck are at high risk for developing oral complications. Because of the risk of osteonecrosis in radiated fields, oral surgery should be performed before radiation treatment begins.

Treatment Goals before Head and Neck Radiation or Chemotherapy

- Begin cancer therapy with a healthy mouth.
- Identify and extract hopeless teeth (7–14 days healing is desired).
- Restore all caries and perform prophylaxis.
- Counsel the patient regarding expected complications of therapy.
- Provide intensive preventive care.

Patient Education

Patient education is an integral part of the pretreatment evaluation and should include a discussion of potential oral complications. To ensure that the patient fully understands what is required, provide detailed instructions on specific oral care practices, such as how and when to brush and floss, how to recognize signs of complications, and other instructions appropriate for the individual.

Advise patients to avoid candy, gum, and soda unless they are sugar free. Likewise, the patient should avoid spicy or acidic foods, tobacco products, and alcohol, including mouthwashes containing alcohol.

Patients should understand that good oral care during cancer treatment contributes to its success. It is very important that the dental team impress on the patient that optimal oral hygiene during treatment, adequate nutrition, and avoiding tobacco and alcohol can prevent or minimize oral complications.

Supplemental Fluoride

Fluoride treatments are essential to protect the teeth of patients treated by radiation therapy directed to the head and neck area. Rinses containing fluoride are not potent enough to prevent dental deterioration. Recommended instead is a high-potency fluoride gel (1.1% neutral pH sodium fluoride) delivered via custom trays. Trays should cover all tooth structures without irritating the gingival or mucosal tissues. Starting several days before radiation therapy begins, patients should use a fluoride gel daily. For patients reluctant to use a tray, a high-potency fluoride gel can be brushed on the teeth following daily brushing and flossing. Most patients with radiation induced salivary gland dysfunction must continue daily fluoride applications for the remainder of their lives.

DENTAL TREATMENT OF PATIENTS AFTER CANCER THERAPY

After Chemotherapy

Once all complications of chemotherapy have resolved, most patients can resume their normal dental care schedule (Figures 9-1 and 9-2). However, if immune function continues to be compromised, determine the patient's hematologic status before initiating any dental treatment or surgery. This is particularly important to remember for patients who have undergone bone marrow transplantation.

A recently detected complication that can develop in individuals treated for advanced-stage cancer involving skeletal metastasis (prostate, breast, lung) and hypercalcemia of malignancy, as well as multiple myeloma, is medication-related osteonecrosis of the jaw (MRONJ) previously known as bisphosphonate related osteonecrosis of the jaws (BRONJ). Bisphosphonates, RANK ligand inhibitor (denosumab) and antiangiogenic medications (e.g., bevacizumab) are associated with MRONJ. Typically,

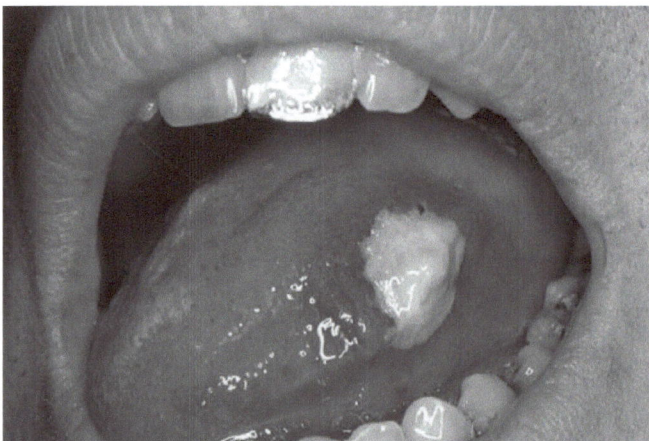

FIGURE 9–1 *Oral mucositis in a post-irradiation head and neck cancer patient.*

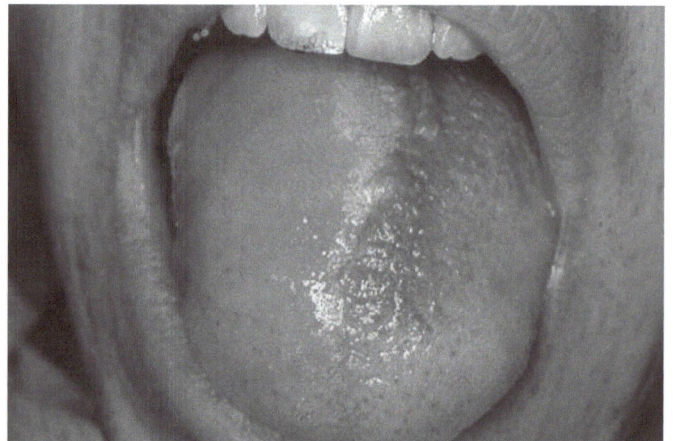

FIGURE 9-2 *Oral mucositis in a post-irradiation head and neck cancer patient.*

TABLE 9–3: Potential Oral Complications from Head and Neck Radiation Therapy	
Complication	**Comment**
Loss of taste/dysgeusia	Taste bud cells are usually capable of repopulating within 4 months following treatment, but some permanent impairment can remain.
Nutritional problems	Oral changes can affect the patient's nutrition and result in inadequate dietary intake. This can be a major cause of morbidity and mortality.
Difficulty with speech and swallowing	Effects can be profound.
Trismus from fibrotic changes to muscles of mastication/TMJ	The full extent of trismus usually becomes evident 3 to 6 months after the end of radiation treatment. Stretching exercises are important during the treatment process to minimize post-treatment trismus.
Hyposalivation/Xerostomia	The degree of xerostomia depends on the fields of radiation. Often xerostomia is permanent and severe, leading to oral discomfort and chronic changes in the oral flora.
Dental caries	Caries can result from hyposalivation and altered oral flora. Dentin hypersensitivity is common.
Osteoradionecrosis	Occurs in 3 to 10% of patients and develops because irradiation diminishes the bone's ability to withstand trauma and avoid infection. The risk does not appear to diminish with time.
TMJ = temporomandibular joint.	

these medications are administered intravenously to decrease the effects of bone metastases by decreasing bone resorption and to interfere with the formation of new blood vessels (bevacizumab) that are important for cancer cell proliferation. In this context, these medications are very useful therapeutic agents.

However, MRONJ is resistant to all current therapy, including hyperbaric oxygen, surgical debridement, antibiotic therapy, and cessation of therapy. Consequently, it is especially important for all patients who are treated with these agents or likely to be treated with them in the future to have a thorough dental evaluation and treatment before cancer therapy begins.

Current Treatment Recommendations for MRONJ
Reports of MRONJ are rapidly increasing in the medical and dental literature. The majority of cases involve intravenous administration of either pamidronate or zoledronic acid. Conservative therapy is recommended with topical and/ or systemic antibiotics as well as appropriate analgesics. Exposed bone can be removed if this can be accomplished conservatively and primary closure obtained. Larger areas of exposed bone can be recontoured and/or covered with vinyl guards or stents and protective coatings. Information on this topic is rapidly evolving, and referral to current

publications is recommended.

After Head and Neck Radiation Therapy
High-dose radiation treatment to the head and neck carries a lifelong risk of osteonecrosis, xerostomia, and dental caries. Lifelong daily fluoride application, good nutrition, and conscientious oral hygiene are especially important for patients with salivary gland dysfunction. A listing of the major complications associated with head and neck radiation therapy appears in Table 9-3.

PREVENTIVE FOCUS

At recall appointments, dental health care workers should thoroughly examine the head and neck area for recurrence of malignancies, especially in patients with oral and head and neck cancers. Dentures may need to be reconstructed if treatment has altered oral tissues. Some individuals can never wear dentures again because of easily irritated alveolar tissues and xerostomia.

Because of the risk of osteonecrosis, principally in the mandible, patients who had a full course of radiation should avoid invasive surgical procedures, including extractions that involve irradiated bone. If an invasive procedure is required, use of antibiotics and hyperbaric oxygen therapy before and after surgery should be considered, and epinephrine should be avoided when local anesthetic is used.

Available Resource For Additional Information

The National Oral Health Information Clearinghouse (NO-HIC; <http://www.nohic.nidcr.nih.gov>; 1-877-216-1019), a service of the National Institute of Dental and Craniofacial Research, maintains a Web site and produces and distributes patient and professional education materials, including fact sheets, brochures, and information packets. NOHIC also sponsors the Oral Health Database, which includes bibliographic citations, abstracts, and availability information for a wide variety of print and audiovisual materials. NOHIC staff provides free custom or standard searches on specific special care topics in oral health. It is an excellent resource.

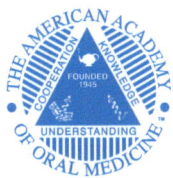

10 Supplemental In-Office Laboratory Testing

Clinical laboratory testing is an essential element of modern medicine (see Table 10-1). For symptomatic patients, laboratory tests often provide the critical information essential for establishing the diagnosis. From a screening perspective, laboratory tests often reveal potentially fatal diseases or conditions, long before the patient becomes symptomatic. Lastly, from a management perspective, laboratory tests are often necessary to monitor the efficacy of prescribed therapeutic protocols. Over the past decade, an explosion of new laboratory tests have been developed and subsequently marketed to both health care professionals and the public. Many purport to be more convenient, to be less invasive, and to provide quicker results than traditional laboratory-based testing schemes. However, these tests add to the cost of health care and often lack validated cost/benefit studies to justify their use. Specific laboratory tests

associated with specific diseases are discussed throughout this monograph and are not repeated here.

Given the fact that many dental patients obtain dental services on a recall driven basis, compared with physician visits, which are often symptom driven, the dentist is in the enviable position of seeing his or her patients more regularly and frequently than his or her medical counterpart. The purpose of this section is to present available in-office tests that may be used in the outpatient dental setting to screen for significant medical conditions, monitor for disease stability, or monitor specific therapeutic interventions. The intent is not to diagnose diseases outside the scope of dental practice but to identify and refer patients at risk for the more common medical conditions affecting the population.

TABLE 10−1: In-Office Tests for Use in Dental Practice			
Test	*Equipment*	*Purpose*	*Normal Range*
Blood pressure/pulse	• Sphygmomanometer and stethoscope for BP • Manual pulse determination (full 60 sec). • Over 180 FDA-approved automatic monitoring machines available	• Identify unrecognized elevations in BP and irregularities in pulse pressure, rate, and rhythm • Monitor efficacy of medical interventions	<120/80 mm Hg
Blood glucose monitoring	• Over 40 FDA-approved blood glucose monitoring systems(OTC type)	• Screen for elevated blood glucose levels. • Monitor status of known diabetes mellitus patient.	FBG = 70–99 mg/dL
	• Hemoglobin A1C levels	• Monitors control over 3 month period	< 5.7 %
INR monitoring	• Several FDA-approved systems	• Verify INR on day of surgery to determine bleeding risk for patients who take coumarin.	INR < 3.5
BP = blood pressure; FBG = fasting blood glucose; INR = international normalized ratio; OTC = over the counter.			

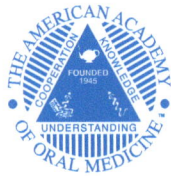

Appendix
The Medical Consultation Process

The medical consultation is an important aspect of the care of medically complex dental patients. It is important for the dental clinician to have an appreciation for the reasons that require medical consultation and the process. Also, the medical consultation process encourages communication between dentists and physicians. Reasons for a medical consultation for dental patients include when the patient is undiagnosed, poorly controlled or you are uncertain of their disease severity, stability or need for therapy. Examples include:

1. The patient's medical condition requires evaluation and possibly therapy. Examples:

   a. Hypertension
   b. Dental erosion that may be secondary to gastric reflux (gastroesophageal reflux disease)
   c. Anemia (pale gingiva, fatigue, white nail beds)

2. Specific medical information or the results of laboratory studies are necessary. Examples:

   a. The results of an echocardiogram
   b. The results of the international normalized ratio (INR)
   c. The results of requested blood studies
   d. The microscopic evaluation of a biopsy
   e. The patient is a poor historian and more information is required regarding the patient's medical or drug history.

3. A request for a change in the patient's medical therapy or prescription regimen is suggested. Examples:

   a. The patient is on one or several drugs that may be causative for drug-induced gingival overgrowth and the dentist requests that the patient's drug regimen be changed.
   b. The patient is being treated with a blood-thinning drug regimen and is scheduled to undergo a dental surgical procedure and the patient's INR is high enough to warrant concern. Therefore, the dentist requests that the patient's drug regimen be adjusted to bring the INR within therapeutic range.

FORMAT FOR A MEDICAL CONSULTATION LETTER BY A DENTIST*

Date: _____

Patient Name: _____

Date of Birth: _____ Age: _____ Sex: _____

Dental Chart Number: _____

_____

To (Physician): _____

Physician's Address: _____

_____

Physician's Phone #: _____

From (Dental Student): _____

Attending Dentist: _____

_____

Patient History: _____

_____

Reason for Consult: _____

_____

Consultant Reply:

                                        Signature of Consultant

                                        _____

* Reproduced with permission from Little JW. Dental management of the medically compromised patient. 6th ed. Elsevier; 2002.

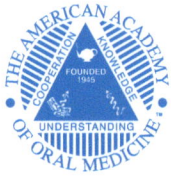

References

- Alataha, D. et al. 2010. "Rheumatoid arthritis classification criteria: an American College of Rheumatology/European League Against Rheumatism collaborative initiative." *Arthritis Rheum* 62(9):2569-81. doi: 10.1002/art.27584

- Copelan E.A. 2006 Apr 27. "Hematopoietic stem-cell transplantation." *N Engl J Med* 354(17):1813-26.

- Feely M.G. 2010. "New and emerging therapies for the treatment of rheumatoid arthritis." *Open Access Rheumatol* 2:35–43. Published online 2010 Jul 24. Dovepress eCollection

- Golla K., J.B. Epstein, and R.J. Cabay. 2004. "Liver disease: current perspectives on medical and dental management." *Oral Surg Oral Med Oral Pathol Oral Radiol Endod* 98(5):516–21.

- Hagner B.F., and A.S. Fouci. 2008. "Disorders of the immune system." edited by Harrison et al. *The principals of internal medicine*, 17th ed., New York, McGraw-Hill.

- Hunter T.M., N.N. Boytsov, X. Zhang, K. Schroeder, K. Michaud, and A.B. Araujo. 2017 Sep. "Prevalence of rheumatoid arthritis in the United States adult population in healthcare claims databases, 2004-2014." *Rheumatol Int* 37(9):1551-1557. doi: 10.1007/s00296-017-3726-1

- Lazarchik D.A., S.J. Filler, and M.P. Winkler. 1995. "Dental evaluation in bone marrow transplantation." *Gen Dent* 143:369–71.

- Little J.W., D.A. Falace, C.S. Miller, and N.L. Rhodus. 2007. *Dental management of the medically compromised patient.* Mosby Elsevier, Publ. Co., St. Louis, MO. 288–91.

- Little J.W., D.A. Falace, C.S. Miller, and N.L. Rhodus. 2007. *Dental management of the medically compromised patient.* Mosby Elsevier, Publ. Co., St. Louis, MO. 319–21.

- Menendez-Jandula B., J.C. Souto, A. Oliver, et al. 2005. "Comparing self-management of oral anticoagulant therapy with clinic management: a randomized trial." *Ann Intern Med* 142:1–10.

- Miller, T.D. 2005. "Mysthena gravis." edited by Kaspar DL and D.R. Harrison. *Harrison's principles of internal medicine*, 16th ed. NY, NY,McGraw-Hill, 766–69.

- Pizzo P.A. 1999. "Fever in immunocompromised patients." *N Engl J Med* 341:893–900.

- Rieken S.E., and G.T. Terezhalmy. 2006. "The pregnant and breast-feeding patient." *Quintessence Int* 37:455–68.

- Saidi R.F., and S. K. Hejazii Kenari. 2014. "Challenges of Organ Shortage for Transplantation: Solutions and Opportunities." *Int J Organ Transplant Med* 5 (3):87–96. Published online 2014 Aug 1. www.ijotm.com

- Selik, R.M., MD, et. al. 2014. *"Revised surveillance case definition for HIV infection – United States, 2014."* CDC Guidelines for the Use of Antiretroviral Agents in Adults and Adolescents Living with HIV, MMWR, Recommendations and Reports. https://www.cdc.gov/mmwr/preview/mmwrhtml/rr6303a1.htm

- Seymour R.A., J.M. Thomason, and A. Nolan. 1997. "Oral lesions in organ transplant patients." *J Oral Pathol Med* 26:297–304.

- Siegel, Rebecca L. MPH, K.D. Miller, MPH; A. Jemal, DVM, PhD. 2018. "Cancer Statistics, 2018" *CA Cancer J Clin* 68:7–30.

- Smolen J.S., D. Aletaha, M. Koeller, M.H. Weisman, and P. Emery. 2007 Dec 1. "New therapies for treatment of rheumatoid arthritis." *Lancet* 370(9602):1861-74

- Sollecito T.P., D. Porter, A. Naji, and A. Pinto. 2007. "Transplant medicine." edited by Greenberg MS, M. Glick, and J. Ship J., *Burket's oral medicine.* 11th ed Hamilton (ON): BC Decker.

- Suresh L., and L. Radfar. 2004. "Pregnancy and lactation." *Oral Surg Oral Med Oral Pathol Oral Radiol Endod* 97:672–82.

- Turner M., and S.R. Aziz. 2002. "Management of the pregnant oral and maxillofacial patient." *J Oral Maxillofac Surg* 60:1479–88.

- U.S. Department of Health and Human Services, Health Resources and Services Administration, 2017 Organ donation statistics.

- U.S. Department of Health and Human Service. Health Resources and Services Administration, 2009 *Annual Report of the U.S. Organ Procurement and Transplantation Network and the Scientific Registry of Transplant Recipients: transplant data 1999 –2008*, Healthcare Systems Bureau, Division of Transplantation, Rockville, MD.

- Worldwide Network for Blood and Marrow Transplantation. Media Fact Sheet: 1 Million Blood Stem Cell Transplants Worldwide. 2013. https://www.wbmt.org/fileadmin/pdf/01_General/2013_WBMT_Annual_Report_ABS_FINAL_to_printer_2014-03-17.pdf

General References
Centers for Disease Control and Prevention
Food and Drug Administration

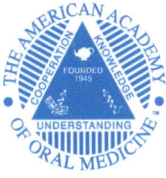

The American Academy of Oral Medicine
2150 N. 107th St., Suite 205
Seattle, Washington 98133
PHONE: (206) 209-5279 · EMAIL: info@aaom.com

Application for AAOM Membership

ELIGIBILITY FOR MEMBERSHIP

1. Nominee for **Regular Membership** shall be a graduate of an accredited Dental School or Medicine School and shall be a member of his/her representative National Society and shall pursue special interest or accomplishment in the field of Oral Medicine.

2. Nominee for **Affiliate Membership** (student) shall be a graduate of an accredited Dental or Medical School and shall be a member of his/her representative National Society and currently in training in a Postdoctoral program.

3. Nominee for **Student Membership** shall be a student currently enrolled in a pre-doctoral program in an accredited dental or medical school. Students are those seeking a DDS, DMD or MD degree.

4. The fiscal year for dues starts January 1.

5. After acceptance into the Academy, Active Membership dues are paid annually and include a subscription to ORAL SURGERY, ORAL MEDICINE, ORAL PATHOLOGY, ORAL RADIOLOGY, and ENDODONTOLOGY.

6. Please see the AAOM website for more membership information and how to apply: www.aaom.com.

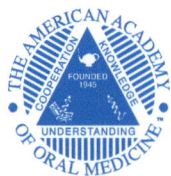